Sobotta/Hammersen

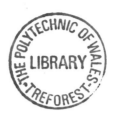

Histology

Color Atlas of Microscopic Anatomy

Frithjof Hammersen, M.D.
Professor and Chairman of the Department of Anatomy
Technical University of Munich

Third edition, revised and enlarged
553 illustrations, most in color

Urban & Schwarzenberg · Baltimore–Munich 1985

Urban & Schwarzenberg, Inc.
7 East Redwood Street
Baltimore, Maryland 21202
U.S.A.

Urban & Schwarzenberg
Pettenkoferstraße 18
D-8000 München 2
Germany

A translation of Sobotta/Hammersen · Histologie, Atlas der Zytologie, Histologie und der mikroskopischen Anatomie.
Urban & Schwarzenberg, München–Wien–Baltimore 1985

Illustration credits:
The figures 116, 209, 210, 250, 256, 261, 265, 266, 284, 286, 288, 294–296, 304–306, 310, 317, 329, 330, 338, 339, 348–350, 354, 367, 387, 388, 396, 398, 410, 411, 417, 422, 428, 472, 473, 483–486, 501–503, 506–510, 515, 516, 531, 533, 538, 539 were taken from: Johannes Sobotta, Atlas und Lehrbuch der Histologie und Mikroskopischen Anatomie.
The figures 152, 153, 158, 272, 273, 289, 345, 439, 440, 449, 452 were taken from: Josef Wallraff, Leitfaden der Histologie des Menschen, 8th edition, Urban & Schwarzenberg, München–Berlin–Wien 1972.
The figures 248, 422 were taken from: Viktor Patzelt, Histologie, 3rd edition, Urban & Schwarzenberg, Wien 1948.

Library of Congress Cataloging in Publication Data

Hammersen, Frithjof.
  Histology, a color atlas of microscopic anatomy.

  Translation of: Histologie, Atlas der mikroskopischen Anatomie. 3. Aufl. 1985.
  At head of title: Sobotta Hammersen.
  Rev. ed. of: Histology, a color atlas of cytology, histology, and microscopic anatomy. 2nd ed., rev. and enl. 1980.
  Many of the drawings were taken from J. Sobotta's Atlas und Lehrbuch der Histologie und mikroskopischen Anatomie.
Includes index.
  1. Histology-Atlases. 2. Anatomy, Human-Atlases.

3. Cytology-Atlases. I. Hammersen, Frithjof. Histology, a color atlas of cytology, histology, and microscopic anatomy. II. Sobotta, Johannes, 1869–1945. Atlas und Lehrbuch der Histologie und mikroskopischen Anatomie. III. Title. [DNLM: 1. Cytology-atlases. 2. Histology-atlases. QS 517.H224a]
QM557.H3313 1985 611'.018 84–29084
ISBN 0-8067-1743-2

Printed in Germany by Kastner & Callwey, München

ISBN 0-8067-1743-2 Baltimore
ISBN 3-541-71743-2 München

87 86 85
6 5 4 3 2 1 0

Preface to the Third Edition

Over the years it has become increasingly apparent that an almost worldwide confusion exists regarding the authorship of this atlas. Dr. Johannes Sobotta (1869–1945), who is generally assumed to be the first author, published in 1902 his *Atlas and Basic Textbook of Human Histology and Microscopic Anatomy,* which contained among others, 80 exquisitely rendered color drawings. Their number increased to almost 400 in the second edition appearing in 1911. By the fourth edition (1929) the illustrations were published in one volume, accompanied by a second volume of elaborate text, and this two-volume set was continued for one more edition, the fifth in 1938. Nearly 40 years elapsed before the first edition of the Sobotta/Hammersen ATLAS appeared, paying tribute to the enormous body of work created by the late Dr. Sobotta by including his name as one of the authors and by reproducing some of the original drawings from his early volumes although drawings may appear somewhat out of place in our modern world.

The first edition of the Sobotta/Hammersen ATLAS was published in 1975 and the second in 1980. The favorable reception of these two editions, and the seemingly appropriate five-year-interval that was established, have given impetus to this new third edition in 1985. Considerable thought has been given to changes, both cosmetic and profound, but author and publisher agree that this book is above all an atlas, and shall remain a collection of illustrative material as complete and as informative as possible. Text is restricted to captions describing the structures seen in the respective illustrations, and deliberately refrains from explanation of detailed functional relationships.

The primary objective of this new edition is to improve the quality of existing illustrations and to add, wherever necessary, new ones. Both of these approaches have been realized by preparing a total of 123 new micrographs (56 in color) for the third edition, either as replacements or additions. This has increased the total number of figures to 553, almost 25% more than are found in the second edition of this ATLAS. The technique of semi-thin sectioning, a routine in electron microscopy, has recently been modified for use in light microscopy, and as such will become increasingly important to high quality histology. We have included a number of illustrations of different tissues prepared by this method, demonstrating the superiority of these sections over those obtained by older, routine techniques.

All of these alterations have been made while continuously keeping in mind the main objective of this book: to present an ATLAS in the truest sense, and one that should be a reliable companion for the practical work with the microscope.

My sincere thanks are due to Mrs. E. Hammersen who, from the first edition onward, has contributed enormously to this ATLAS in every respect. I am particularly obliged to my friend John G. Simpson, MB, ChB, PhD, MRCPath, Senior Lecturer in

Pathology, University of Aberdeen, Scotland, for the enormous body of work and his never-ceasing patience when correcting the English style of my manuscript. Thanks are also due to Mrs. A. Sattelmair, Mrs. G. Terfloth, and Mrs. B. Zschiesche, whose technical skills are mirrored in several micrographs. I am also indebted to Mrs. E. Haussmann for secretarial help. To Mrs. B. Ruppel, together with whom the new diagrams (Figs. 1, 2, 182, and 366) were developed, I owe particular thanks. It was a pleasure to work with her and see her transform our ideas into reality.

I am also grateful to my co-workers Dr. M. I. Behrens, Dr. U. Herrmann, Dr. P. Oldenbüttel, and Dr. A. Reinhardt, who carefully read the galley proofs and made valuable contributions coming from their experience with our students.

Furthermore, it is a pleasure to express my thanks and appreciation not only to the publisher, Mr. Michael Urban, who met my wishes with great understanding and most generous cooperation, but also to his technical staff who converted my manuscript into this ATLAS. To all of them I express my sincere gratitude.

Finally, it is hoped that we have succeeded in our shared effort to improve this Third Edition in such a way that it serves the student like Ariadne's thread, as a reliable guide that leads safely through the initially confusing labyrinth of cytologic and histologic structures. This is the essential goal around which the Sobotta/Hammersen ATLAS has been conceived.

Munich, January 1985   *Frithjof Hammersen*

Contents

Contents

Contents

How to Use this Book

This chapter is new to the 3rd edition of Sobotta/Hammersen ATLAS, and has been conceived as a special aid to the reader. Both the author and the publisher hope that, by careful attention to the points listed below, optimal use of this text can be made.

1. The Preface has been written, in part, as a history of the Sobotta/Hammersen ATLAS, and discusses the intentions of the author as well as explains the book's design and organization.

2. At the end of the ATLAS 15 tables summarize a variety of topics such as staining properties of the most common histologic stains, classification of the various components of connective tissue, or numerous types of histologic fibers which, regardless of their profound structural differences, are collectively referred to as "fibers."

3. Before studying a light or electron micrograph, it is important to read its caption carefully; each describes as accurately as possible the structures to be seen in the micrograph. In order to encourage this, the number of labels on each illustration has been kept to a minimum. The captions provide the tools to enable the student to identify the various structural components of cells and tissues by their characteristic features instead of simply following leader lines.

4. This ATLAS is not meant to replace a comprehensive textbook of histology, but rather to enhance and supplement text use. It is highly recommended that the student begins with careful reading of the respective chapter in the textbook before referring to the ATLAS, and not vice versa.

5. This ATLAS has been designed as a visual guide to the often confusing multitude of cytologic and histologic details seen in the large number of specimens usually demonstrated in a course of normal histology. Therefore, the first priority has been given to describing structures as precisely as possible. Description of functional implication is given far less importance and only occasionally appears.

6. Included in the captions are those criteria that allow for clear distinction between certain tissues and organs which, because of their structural similarity, may be confused easily; e.g., the lactating mammary gland and the prostate gland. These criteria are also summarized according to the respective tissues and organs in tables appearing at the end of the book.

7. In order to identify structural details more easily, it may be helpful to view the micrographs through a simple magnifying glass; the electron micrographs, particularly, will be enhanced.

8. We did not strive for ultimate perfection in every case because we feel that students should not get accustomed to the most beautiful specimens available each coming from another highly specialized laboratory. Students should be confronted, instead, with specimens displaying a technical quality such as can be achieved by a routine laboratory for light and electron microscopy.

Fundamentals of Histologic Techniques

In courses of normal and pathologic histology the student is usually confronted with thin stained sections of tissues and organs that are mounted under a cover slip to provide permanent preparations. In order to interpret these tissue slices correctly and critically, e.g., to be aware of artifacts, the student should be familiar with the fundamentals of histologic techniques.

Without the use of special optical equipment such as phase or interference contrast microscopes, living cells and tissues are almost invisible because of the minimal refraction differences existing among the various cellular and tissue constituents. The living tissues and organs are, therefore, subjected to defined procedures to obtain from them thin stained slices which usually exhibit high contrast. These procedures consist mainly of the following consecutive steps (see also Figs. 1 and 2).

Fixation

The fixation should serve at least three different functions:

1. As good a preservation of the tissue as possible in order to stabilize its constituents in an almost *in vivo* condition. Since this is only achievable within certain limits because of the high water content of living materials, a perfect chemical fixative does not exist.

2. An increase in the hardness of the tissue to improve the ease with which it can be cut into thin slices.

3. The killing of all bacteria and other infective agents present in the tissue.

Many of our fixatives, of which the most common is a neutral 4% solution of formaldehyde, are strong precipitants of proteins (e.g., picric acid and mercury bichloride); and hence they coagulate the constituents of cells and tissues. This severe denaturation can be avoided by using a 2.5% solution of glutaraldehyde in a defined buffer (pH 7.4), which is administered – if possible – by vascular perfusion of the organ itself or of an entire experimental animal. This is the most commonly used fixation technique for electron microscopy (see also Figs. 1 and 2).

Embedding

In order to obtain sufficiently thin sections (ca. $10\,\mu$m for routine light and ca. 50 nm = 500 Å for electron microscopy) from the fixed and thereby already hardened pieces of tissue, specially designed cutting devices are used (microtomes for light and ultramicrotomes for electron microscopy); and the specimen must be embedded in a solidifying material which can then be cut. As these embedding materials are not soluble in water, it must be removed by placing the tissue step by step through a series of graded alcohol or acetone. This dehydration procedure should be carried out very carefully yet thoroughly, so that finally all the water is removed and is replaced by 100% alcohol or acetone. Thereby the tissue not only becomes additionally hardened, but all its components soluble in alcohol or acetone, e.g., lipids, are dissolved and removed (cf. Figs. 55, 127). During this step of the preparation a particularly great number of artifacts, such as shrinkage (cf. Fig. 16) or disruption of the tissue (cf. Fig. 18), may occur. Paraffin wax is still the most common of embedding materials for light microscopy, whereas various types of polymerizing resins like Epon, Araldite and others are used in electron microscopy (cf. Figs. 1, 2).

A particularly good preservation of cellular structures can be achieved by placing the freshly obtained tissue into liquid nitrogen and then cutting these frozen specimens with a special cryomicrotome, thereby avoiding the disadvantages of the process of dehydration such as shrinkage and the dissolution of lipids (cf. Fig. 126).

Staining

Paraffin sections prepared as described above are firmly attached to glass slides, and these are transferred into staining solutions to increase the contrast among the various tissue ingredients. Since most of these staining solutions are aqueous in nature, it is necessary to remove the paraffin by placing the section into an appropriate solvent (a clearing agent, e.g., xylol). The solvent must be removed by absolute alcohol, and then the section is transferred into a series of graded alcohol until it is finally placed in water. This is the reverse of the process employed in dehydrating the tissue. When exposed to the staining solutions or mixtures of them, the various tissue constituents take on different colors with different intensities, and this property is greatly influenced by the pH of the staining solution. Besides a series of routine stainings

1

Steps in preparing sections for light microscopy

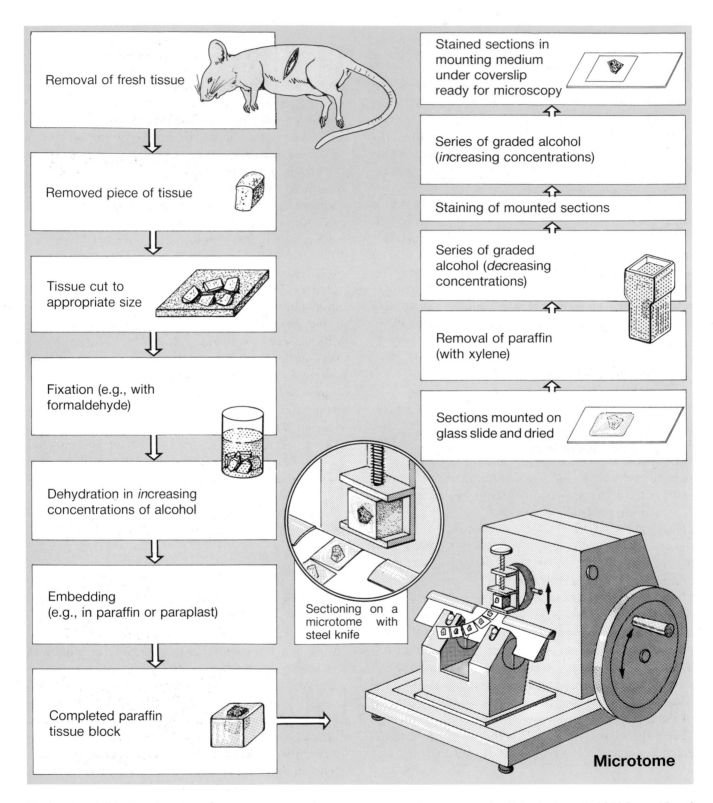

Fig. 1. Schematic drawing and flow chart of the successive steps necessary to prepare a stained histologic section (thickness 10 μm) ready for light microscopic analysis (drawing by Mrs. B. Ruppel, Munich, FRG).

Steps in preparing sections for electron microscopy

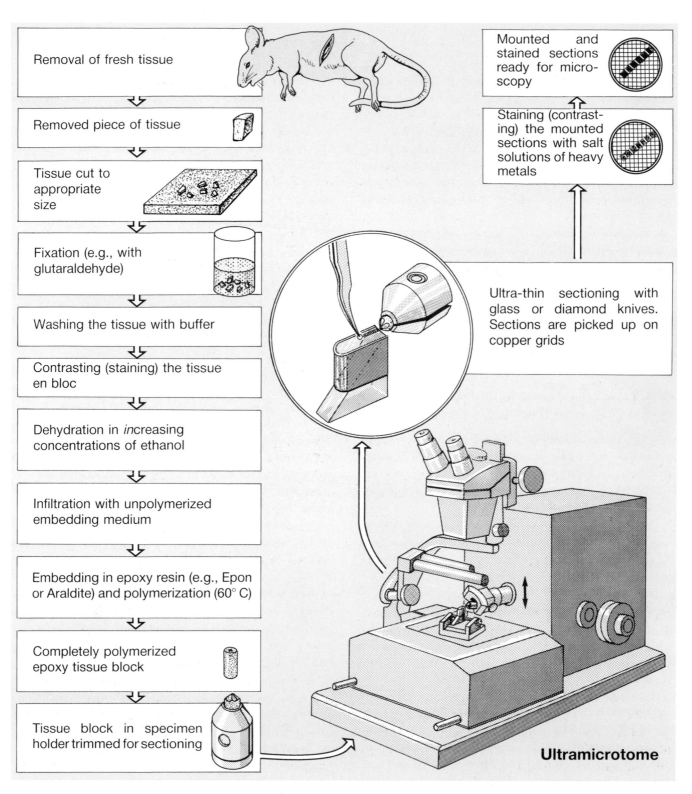

Fig. 2. Schematic drawing and flow chart of the successive steps necessary to prepare ultra-thin sections (thickness 50 nm) ready for electron microscopic analysis from a freshly obtained piece of tissue (drawing by Mrs. B. Ruppel, Munich, FRG).

3

How to handle histologic specimens and how to interprete their images

(Figs. 5–12), a great number of special procedures have been developed, among which the so-called histo-topo-chemical methods play a pivotal role in modern histology. These methods allow for a clear identification of a great variety of chemically defined substances such as glycogen, enzymes, lipids, mucopolysaccharides and others at their actual location within cells and tissues, thereby providing much better insight into the biological dynamics of cells.

In electron microscopy, ca. 50 nm (500 Å) thick, so-called ultra-thin sections (mean square area: 0.25 mm²) are placed on circular copper grids (diameter 3 mm) and are then transferred into the electron beam of the microscope by means of a specially designed specimen holder. The electron microscopic image of such a section is studied on a fluorescent screen, and it can be documented photographically.

A Few Remarks to Improve the Interpretation and Identification (Differential Diagnosis) of Histologic Sections

In order to achieve a critical estimate of what a histologic section can and cannot prove and how the various structures seen in a section may be interpreted correctly, the student should always be aware of a few very simple, yet often neglected facts:

1. The histologic section can only provide a sort of "snapshot" produced by fixation from the continuously changing, dynamic processes occurring in living cells and tissues.

2. The majority of all histologic sections represent a very thin slice of a small piece from a comparably large organ, e.g., the human liver. Due to the often inhomogeneous distribution of certain structures or pathologic processes these cannot be found in every section yet this does not prove that they do not exist.

3. Histologic section viewed at a single level of focus is essentially a two-dimensional representation of three-dimensional cells and tissues. To visualize the minute third dimension in paraffin sections (= thickness of section), the microscope objective should be focused progressively from the upper surface of the section down to its bottom. Immediate conclusions as to the true three-dimensional configuration of cells, tissues, and their ingredients can be drawn from a single section only in a

very few exceptional cases and even then caution is necessary. This may be illustrated with the following simple examples:

a) Circular profiles, irrespective of whether they are of light or electron microscopic dimensions, could represent transverse sections through cylinders, globules, ellipsoids or cones. If all the profiles seen in one section are of identical size then this would point to cross-sectioned cylinders rather than to any other configuration, because it is not very probable that, e.g., all globules or cones would have been cut at the same level of their circumferences.

b) The occurrence of two nuclei within the same cell is no proof at all that this cell is actually binucleated. In most cases this is due to sections through a bent or curved nucleus (cf. Figs. 24, 233), and an apparent "hole" within a nucleus is nothing but a deep cross-sectioned nuclear indentation.

c) The easiest way to improve the ability to think in three dimensions – and this is essential to interpret histologic sections correctly – is to imagine sections cut in variant planes through familiar three-dimensional objects, or even actually to perform such sections (cf. Fig. 3). If you cut a hardboiled egg transversely at the site of its two poles (cf. Fig. 3c) or cut its periphery lengthwise, none of these three sections will show the yolk, but this does not prove that it does not exist. Cross- and longitudinal sections through a straight or curved tube (Figs. 3a, b) may display very different appearances, depending on where and how the sections are cut; and a nearly identical situation may be expected if biological tubes like blood vessels or urinary tubules are involved (cf. Figs. 366, 376–378). Finally, an orange, at least comparable to a secretory unit (acinus) of an exocrine gland like the parotid gland, can appear very different if sectioned in different planes (Fig. 3d). Many more such simple examples can be found, but these few should stand for the rest of them, as a *pars pro toto,* to illustrate how to develop three-dimensional images from histologic sections, which are predominantly two-dimensional objects.

4. To identify an unknown histologic specimen with certainty and to establish a well-founded differential diagnosis, a few basic rules should be followed that guarantee a systematic procedure in every case.

a) A histologic section should always be inspected thoroughly with the naked eye, because certain organs

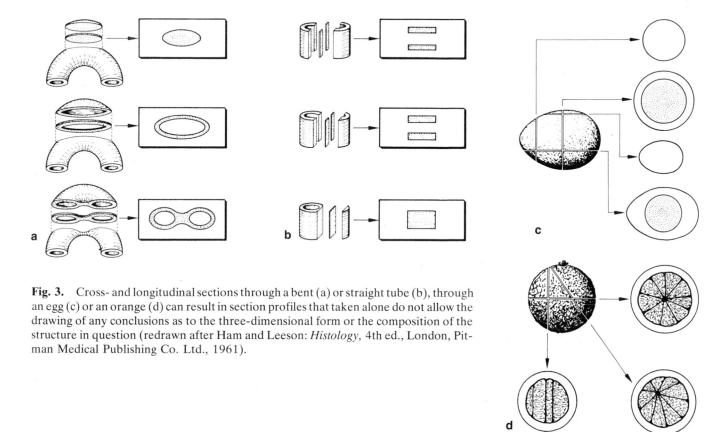

Fig. 3. Cross- and longitudinal sections through a bent (a) or straight tube (b), through an egg (c) or an orange (d) can result in section profiles that taken alone do not allow the drawing of any conclusions as to the three-dimensional form or the composition of the structure in question (redrawn after Ham and Leeson: *Histology,* 4th ed., London, Pitman Medical Publishing Co. Ltd., 1961).

may be definitely identified if cut in a typical plane like the hypophysis in a midsagittal section (Fig. 449) or a cross-sectioned adrenal gland (Fig. 465).

b) This should be followed by an inspection with a simple magnifying glass or, if not available, with the *lowest power* objective of the microscope. During this step pay particular attention to the following: Is the section organized into definite layers (corresponding to a "cortex" and a "medulla")? Does a fibrous capsule exist? Can a lumen be found? Does the section contain very differently colored areas, or does it show regular folds of its surface?

c) Then the entire section has to be observed with the lowest power objective, i.e., each of its free margins must have been seen. Otherwise one of the most essential questions arising in this context, whether the histologic section displays an epithelium, cannot be definitely decided. If the answer is "yes", then first of all the epithelium must be carefully identified, because already this guides further considerations in a certain direction, as shown with the following example. If a "simple columnar epithelium" has been found, this section could theoretically come from either the digestive canal or from the inner female reproductive organs (uterine tube or uterus). To substantiate the first of these two possibilities, one looks for the characteristic layering of the wall as found in all parts of the digestive tube (cf. Fig. 310). If this can be confirmed, then the section originates with certainty from either the stomach or from the intestinal canal. (For further diagnostic procedures, see Table 13.) In case this typical wall texture is absent, then the section has either been obtained from the gallbladder or the second of the two preliminary diagnoses is true. To decide this (1) search for kinocilia that are characteristic for uterine mucosa and the fallopian tube at defined menstrual stages and (2) relate this feature to the rest of structures, e.g., the occurrence of intensely branched mucosal folds (uterine tube, Fig. 428) or epithelial invaginations as to

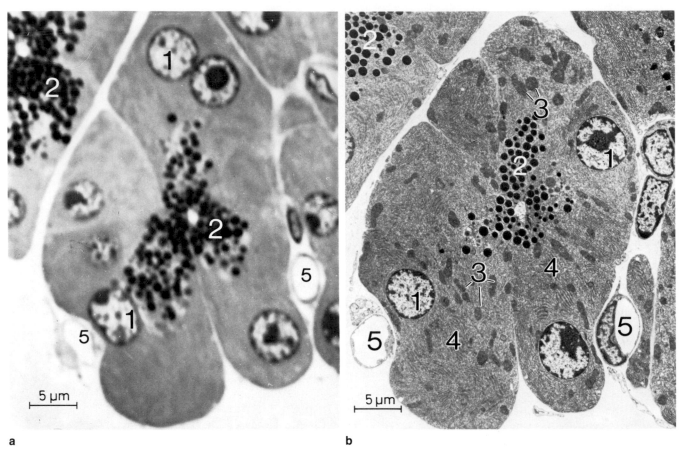

a   b

Fig. 4. A light (**a**) and an electron micrograph (**b**) of the same serous acinus from rat salivary gland to illustrate the difference between magnification and resolution. Although both photographs have the same final magnification of × 2,500, the light microscopic picture reveals nothing except the nuclei (**1**), the secretory granules (**2**) and the acinar lumen, but no structural details of the remaining cytoplasm.
By contrast, the electron microscopic picture taken with higher primary resolving power displays in addition several cytoplasmic organelles like mitochondria (**3**) and an abundance of orderly arrayed cisternae of the rough endoplasmic reticulum (**4**). The nuclear chromatic material also stands out more clearly as do other structures like, e.g., the surrounding capillaries (**5**).

form simple glands (uterine mucosa, Fig. 434) or the existence of low mucosal folds that anastomose with one another (gallbladder, Fig. 327).
d) These consecutive steps in identifying a histologic specimen can almost always be performed, at least in 95% of all cases, with the lowest power or at most with a medium power objective. If the specimen is not identified with these, it will never be identified at all. This may also be demonstrated with a simple example: To distinguish the various "serous" glands from one another (cf. Table 12, and Figs. 307–309), the pancreas must be included in these considerations. Since the otherwise so characteristic "islets" are very rare in the head region and in the un-

cinate process, or are even entirely lacking in these areas, the inexperienced student thinks the "centro-acinar cells" to be the other most reliable criterion to differentiate the pancreas from the rest of the serous glands. Yet for a beginner it is far more difficult to identify the centro-acinar cells as such than to evaluate the most simplest but much safer criterion, namely, the complete absence of salivary (striated) ducts from the exocrine pancreas. But the student searching with the highest power objective for centro-acinar cells must inevitably overlook this characteristic feature due to the very small microscopic field related to high power objectives, and hence the pancreas will not be correctly identified.

Cytology

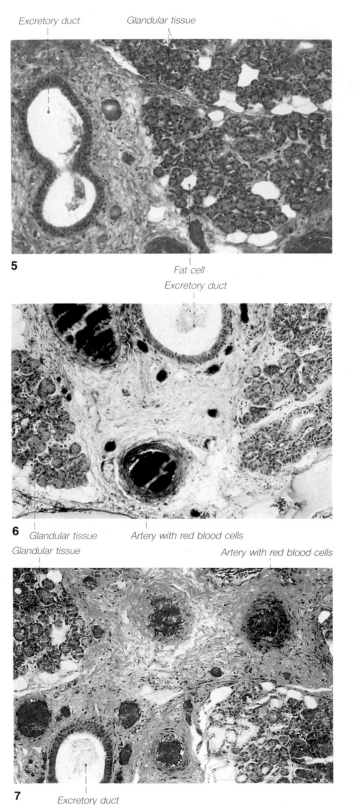

5

Excretory duct   *Glandular tissue*

Fat cell

Excretory duct

6   *Glandular tissue*   *Artery with red blood cells*

Glandular tissue   *Artery with red blood cells*

7   *Excretory duct*

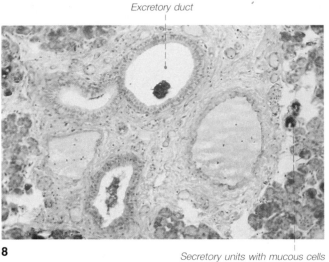

Excretory duct

8   *Secretory units with mucous cells*

Figures 5 to 12 serve as a comparison of eight common staining procedures used here on sections of the same specimen (human submandibular gland). All figures are shown at the same magnification: × 100. For further details see Table 1.

Fig. 5. Hematoxylin-eosin staining, in short: HE or H & E, is by far the most common and most frequently employed technique in normal and pathologic histology.

Fig. 6. Iron hematoxylin according to Heidenhain is a stain formerly widely used in normal histology to demonstrate finer cytologic details like mitochondria, centrioles and tonofibrils at the level of light microscopy (cf. also Figs. 40, 478).

Fig. 7. Trichrome staining according to Masson (also known in a modification as Masson-Goldner) has the advantage of staining collagenous fibers distinctly (green) from all cytoplasmic components (purplish-red).

Fig. 8. PAS-staining (abbreviation for *p*eriodic-*a*cid-*S*chiff-reaction) selectively colors glycogen as well as muco- and glycoproteins and some of glucosaminoglycans in purplish tint (clearly seen within the mucus-secreting cells of the acini).

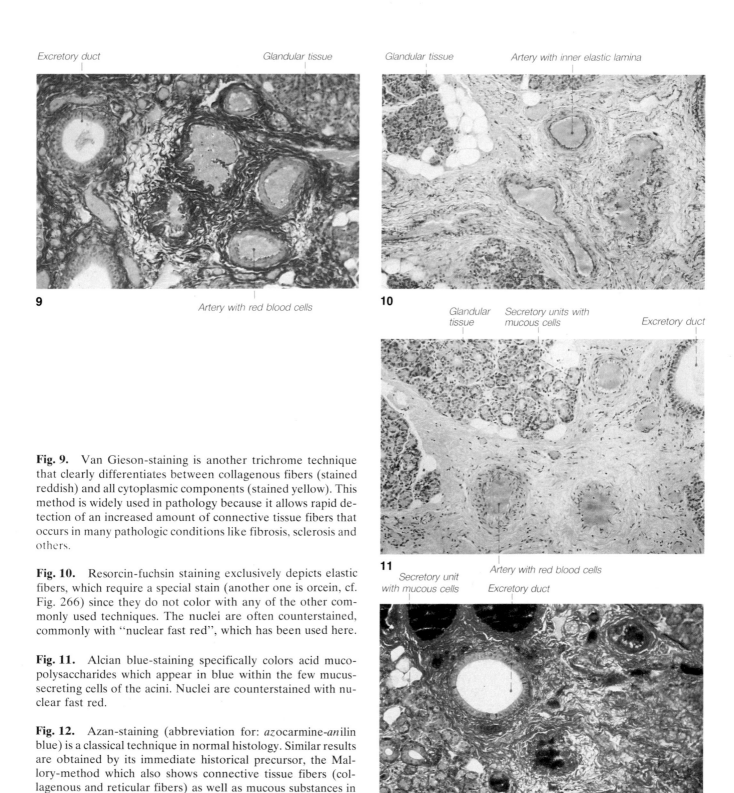

Excretory duct   *Glandular tissue*

9

Artery with red blood cells

Glandular tissue   *Artery with inner elastic lamina*

10

Glandular tissue   *Secretory units with mucous cells*   *Excretory duct*

11   *Artery with red blood cells*

Secretory unit with mucous cells   *Excretory duct*

12

Glandular tissue

Fig. 9. Van Gieson-staining is another trichrome technique that clearly differentiates between collagenous fibers (stained reddish) and all cytoplasmic components (stained yellow). This method is widely used in pathology because it allows rapid detection of an increased amount of connective tissue fibers that occurs in many pathologic conditions like fibrosis, sclerosis and others.

Fig. 10. Resorcin-fuchsin staining exclusively depicts elastic fibers, which require a special stain (another one is orcein, cf. Fig. 266) since they do not color with any of the other commonly used techniques. The nuclei are often counterstained, commonly with "nuclear fast red", which has been used here.

Fig. 11. Alcian blue-staining specifically colors acid mucopolysaccharides which appear in blue within the few mucus-secreting cells of the acini. Nuclei are counterstained with nuclear fast red.

Fig. 12. Azan-staining (abbreviation for: *az*ocarmine-*an*ilin blue) is a classical technique in normal histology. Similar results are obtained by its immediate historical precursor, the Mallory-method which also shows connective tissue fibers (collagenous and reticular fibers) as well as mucous substances in various shades of blue and thereby distinctly different from the reddish-stained nuclei and cytoplasmic components.

Cytology – Artifacts

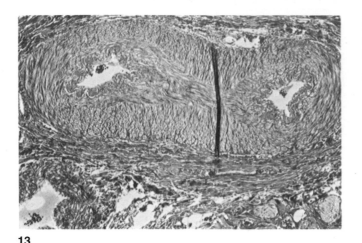

13

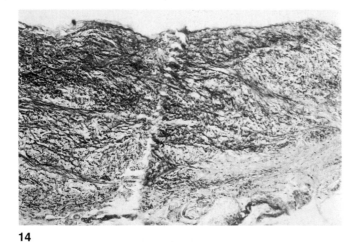

14

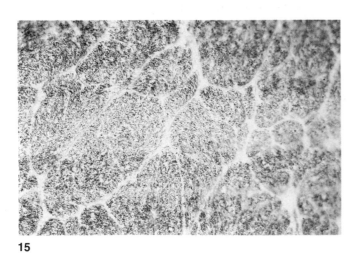

15

A collection of artifacts due to various technical imperfections. One of the most common is caused by shrinkage during the dehydration process and depends mainly on the differing water content of tissues.

Fig. 13. Inadequate stretching of the section on the slide results in folds that are easily recognized since they appear as darker stained strands (artery in the capsule of a human seminal vesicle). The folds, caused by not warming the paraffin carefully, give a rough estimate of the thickness of the section. The connective tissue in the lower part of the picture shows cracks and clefts. Mallory-azan staining. Magnification 75×.

Fig. 14. Scratch in a section caused by a nick in the microtome knife (human aortic valve). Resorcin-fuchsin staining. Magnification 100×.

Fig. 15. Irregular section thickness due to chattering of the knife causes differences in staining intensity, seen here as a lighter stained band crossing the section (human spinal cord). Weigert's stain for myelin. Magnification 60×.

A collection of artifacts due to various technical imperfections. One of the most common is caused by shrinkage during the dehydration process and depends mainly on the differing water content of tissue.

Artificial space caused by shrinkage   Villus

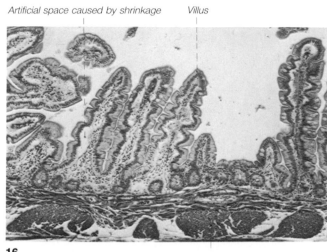

16

Muscularis externa

Fig. 16. Extensive shrinkage clefts occurring between the epithelium and underlying lamina propria of jejunal villi (human jejunum). Note the same artifact between muscle fibers of the muscularis externa and the adjacent connective tissue. Mallory-azan staining. Magnification 75×.

Fixative precipitate

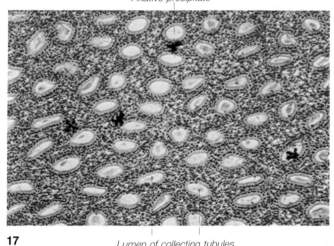

17

Lumen of collecting tubules

Fig. 17. Quite often various fixatives, e.g., formalin, sublimate, if not completely removed, can form crystalline precipitates, seen here as irregularly shaped black structures (rabbit renal papilla). H & E staining. Magnification 75×.

Artificial disruption of muscle fibers

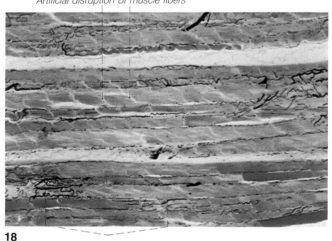

18

Injected blood vessels

Fig. 18. If there is excessive hardening, e.g., by exposing the specimen too long to benzene or benzene-paraffin during the embedding procedure, the tissue becomes friable and sectioning results in cracks (canine rectus femoris muscle, blood vessels injected with ink). H & E staining. Magnification 75×.

Nucleolus Nucleus of satellite cell

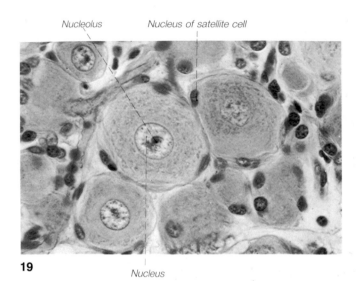

19

Nucleus

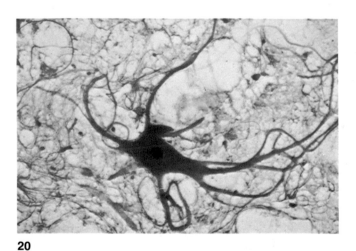

20

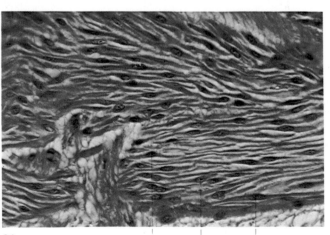

21   Nuclei of spindle-shaped smooth muscle cells

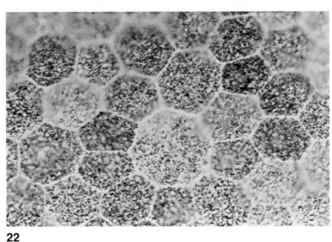

22

Fig. 19. Spinal ganglion cells. Note the characteristic eye-like appearance of these cells due to their round nuclei with prominent nucleoli. The flat nuclei attached to the ganglion cell surfaces belong to satellite cells, a type of peripheral glial cell. Preparations of ganglion cells or of primary ovarian follicles are often used to demonstrate general cellular features. Mallory-azan staining. Magnification 600×.

Fig. 20. Multipolar motor neuron of the bovine spinal cord. This cell was isolated by maceration and then stained and mounted whole as a squash preparation to demonstrate all of its extensions. With routine sectioning techniques most of these cell processes would be cut off, leaving only a few in the plane of the section. Acid fuchsin staining. Magnification 240×.

Fig. 21. Longitudinal section of smooth muscle (rabbit gallbladder), the cells arrayed like a school of fish. Note the elliptical nuclei, which are often difficult to distinguish from the cytoplasm. Hematoxylin and chromotrop staining. Magnification 380×.

Fig. 22. Unstained spread ("Häutchen" preparation) of the isolated eye pigment epithelium (horse) demonstrating the hexagonal outline of these cells. The pigment is seen as granules distributed homogeneously in the cyptoplasm. Magnification 600×.

12

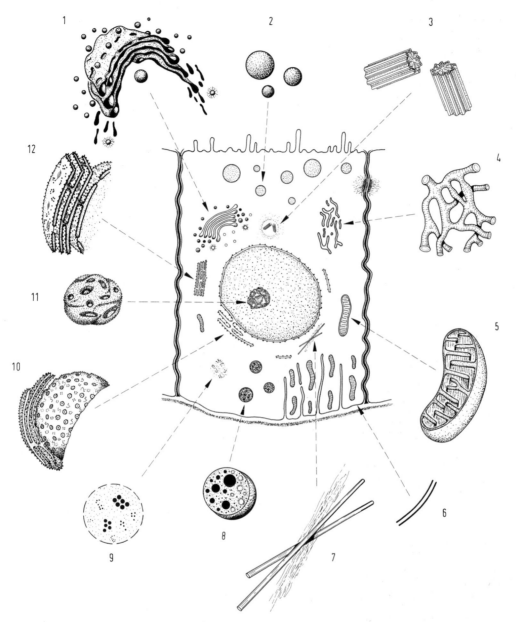

Fig. 23. Schematic representation of a eukaryotic cell with its major organelles, cytoplasmic constituents, and surface specializations (redrawn and extensively modified after Bloom and Fawcett: *Textbook of Histology,* 10th ed., Philadelphia–London–Toronto, W. B. Saunders Co., 1975). Because conventional electron micrographs only show a two-dimensional view of these structures they are depicted here in enlarged three-dimensional fashion. Due to the space available, the relative proportions of the structures have been disregarded. **1** Golgi complex (= Golgi apparatus) with saccules, vesicles, coated vesicles and vacuoles; **2** Secretion granules; **3** A pair of centrioles (= diplosome); **4** Smooth endoplasmic reticulum (SER); **5** Mitochondrion, crista-type; **6** Cell membrane (plasmalemma); **7** Microtubules and filaments; **8** Lysosome; **9** Glycogen particles and polyribosomes; **10** Nucleus seen *en face* with its pores and surrounding cisternae of rough endoplasmic reticulum; **11** Nucleolus with nucleolonema; **12** Highly ordered stacks of cisternae of rough endoplasmic reticulum (RER). They can be recognized in light microscopy as basophilic material termed ergastoplasm (cf. Fig. 29).

The free (upper) surface of the cell bears several irregular microvilli and the basal (lower) cell membrane exhibits several regular deep infoldings.

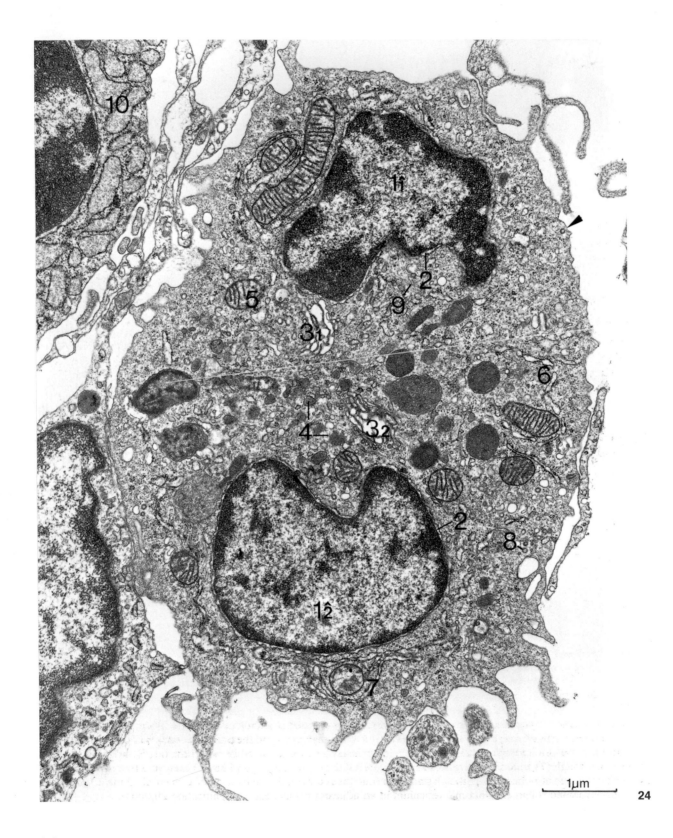

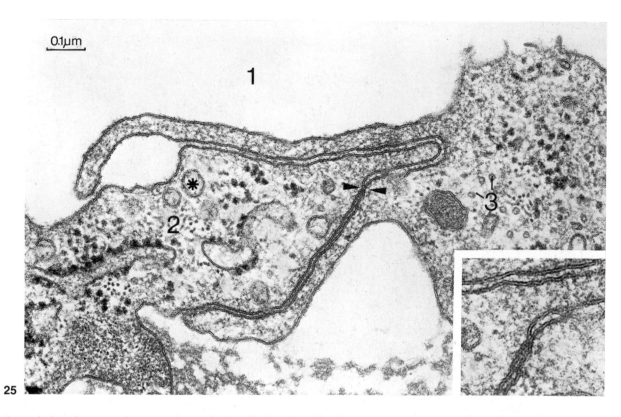

Fig. 25. High resolution electron microscopy is required to disclose the trilaminar appearance of the **cell membrane** and its derivatives such as micropinocytotic vesicles (✳). At the interface of these two endothelial cells from the coronary artery of a pig there is a point-like fusion (► ◄) of the outer layers of the two cell membranes. A close-up of this fusion or macula occludens is shown in the inset. **1** Vascular lumen; **2** Filaments in cross-section; **3** Microtubules in cross-section. Magnification 100,000 × and 185,000 ×.

Fig. 24. Macrophage (histiocyte) from mouse connective tissue to illustrate **normal cellular components.** The nucleus is cut twice in this section (1_1, 1_2) due to its curved shape. The outer of the two nuclear membranes and the perinuclear space (**2**) can be identified. Immediately adjacent to two Golgi complexes (3_1, 3_2) are several primary lysosomes (**4**), while mitochondria (**5**) and small cisternae of both smooth (**6**) and rough (**7**) endoplasmic reticulum are scattered throughout the cytoplasm. Coated vesicles originating from the Golgi complex can be seen at ► fusing with the plasmalemma and thus contributing to its continued renewal. **9** Intracytoplasmic filaments; **10** Well-developed rough endoplasmic reticulum in an adjacent plasma cell. Magnification 20,000 ×.

Electron microscopy – Cell membrane and its specializations

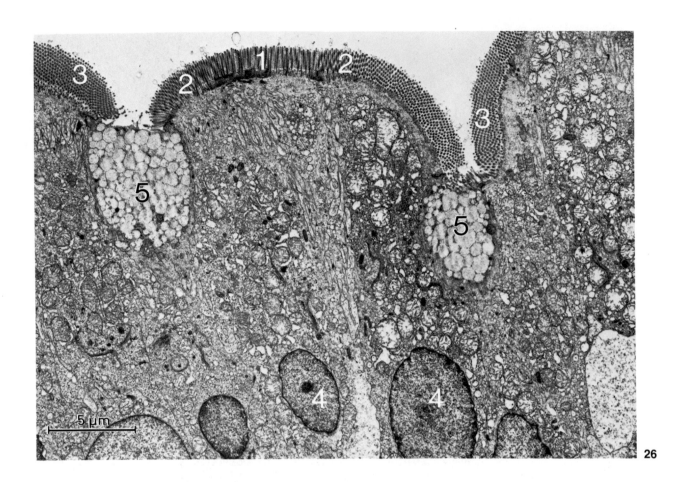

26

Fig. 26. Low-power electron micrograph of intestinal columnar epithelium from rat duodenum to illustrate one of the stable surface specializations of cell membranes, i.e. **microvilli** in longitudinal (**1**), oblique (**2**), and cross-section (**3**); **4** = nucleus; **5** = Goblet cell. For details see Figure 27. Magnification 4,500 ×.

Fig. 27a, b. **Microvilli** of the intestinal epithelium in longitudinal and cross section (rat jejunum). These finger-like projections are very uniform in shape and size (mean length 0.9 μm, mean diameter 0.1 μm) and show a very regular close spacing over the entire cell surface. Together they form the striated or brush border seen by light microscopy (see Fig. 91). Because of the high resolution of these micrographs, both the trilaminar structure of the cell membrane and the fine parallel filaments situated in the core of the microvilli are clearly visible. The filaments are possibly contractile and merge in a perpendicularly oriented filamentous sheet, the terminal web (**1**), itself spread parallel and close to the cell surface. Magnification 78,000 × and 72,000 ×.

Fig. 28. Particularly well-developed **basal labyrinth** in an epithelial cell from the proximal convoluted renal tubule (rat). The deep plasmalemmal infoldings form a complex system of irregular clefts bordering on narrow cytoplasmic septa that contain many slender elongated mitochondria (**1**). Adjacent to the basal lamina, the cytoplasmic septa show ill-defined condensations (▸) corresponding to poorly differentiated hemidesmosomes (see also Fig. 63b). Magnification 18,000 ×.

16

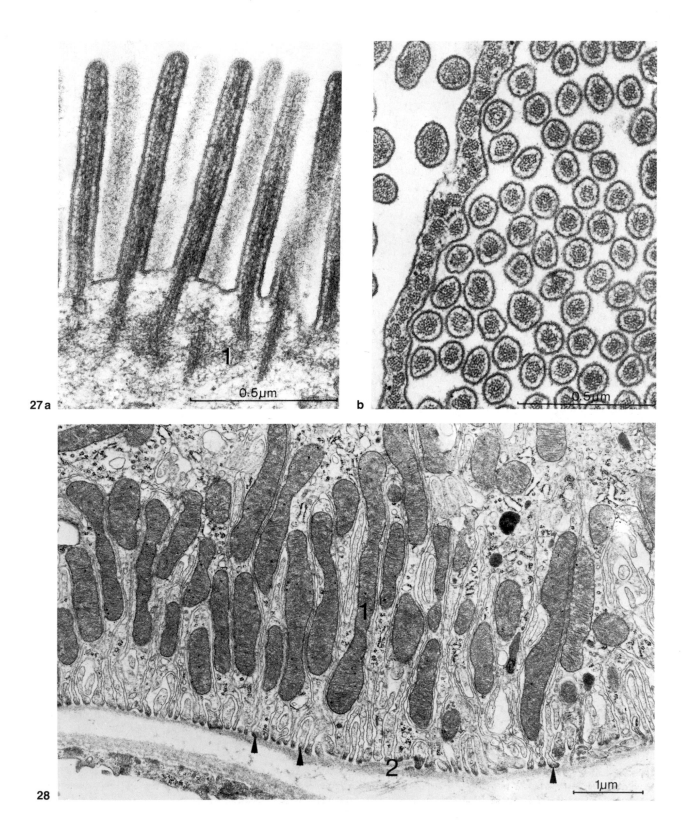

27 a

0.5 μm

b

0.5 μm

28

1 μm

Light microscopy – Ergastoplasm and Golgi complex

Ergastoplasm

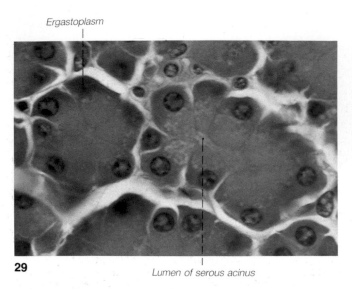

29

Lumen of serous acinus

Nucleus of ganglion cell with prominent nucleolus

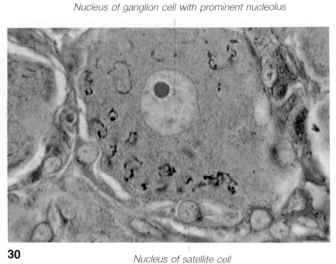

30

Nucleus of satellite cell

Fig. 29. Acini of a canine exocrine pancreas showing marked basophilia of the basal parts of the secretory cells. This staining property is due to the large amounts of RNA present in the ribosomes of the **ergastoplasm** (see also Figs. 31, 35). H & E staining. Magnification 960×.

Fig. 30. Neurons from a feline spinal ganglion with the **Golgi complexes** showing as ribbon-shaped structures. Kolatschev's osmium technique with safranin counterstaining of nuclei and nucleoli. Magnification 960×.

Fig. 31. Part of an acinus from a rat exocrine pancreas. In this low-power electron micrograph the **ergastoplasm** (RER) (**1**) appears as a system of electron-dense (due to the attached ribosomes) membranes that enclose essentially parallel, slightly curved spaces of varying width. **2** Nucleus; **3** Secretory granules. Magnification 12,500×.

Fig. 32. Low-power electron micrograph of two **Golgi complexes** (**1**) in an epithelial cell of a cat salivary gland duct. Each of these complexes corresponds approximately to one of the ribbon- or hook-shaped structures seen with the light microscope after osmication as in Figure 30. **2** Nucleus; **3** Mitochondrion; **4** Intercellular space with desmosomes (►). Magnification 32,000×.

18

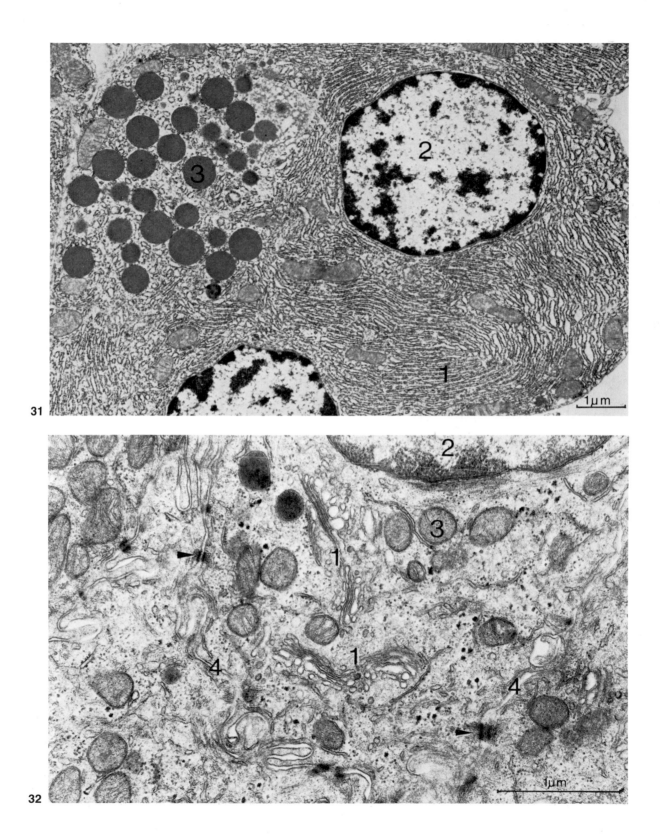

31

32

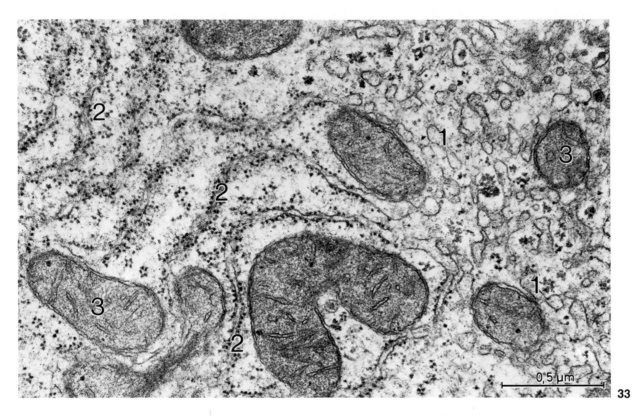

Fig. 33. Part of a rat liver cell (hepatocyte) that contains granular or **rough endoplasmic reticulum** (RER) on the left (**2**) and agranular or **smooth** *ER* (SER) on the right (**1**). The SER lacks ribosomal studding and appears here in the form of elongated oval membrane profiles. **3** Mitochondrion. Magnification 53,000×.

Fig. 34. Well-developed **smooth endoplasmic reticulum** in the apical part of an epithelial cell from mouse trachea, showing its tube-shaped elements at →. **1** Mitochondrion; **2** Microperoxisome. Magnification 44,000×.

Fig. 35. **Ergastoplasm** in a rat exocrine pancreatic cell. The ergastoplasm consists of stacks of rough endoplasmic reticulum, the parallel membranes of which are heavily studded with ribosomes and enclose narrow elongated cavities (cisternae), occasionally showing vacuolar dilatations at their free edges (✳). A well-developed RER forming an ergastoplasm always indicates a high rate of protein synthesis. The products of this activity are not required for cell metabolism, but serve as "export proteins" used in the formation of secretory products, intercellular substances, etc. **1** Nucleus. Magnification 38,000×.

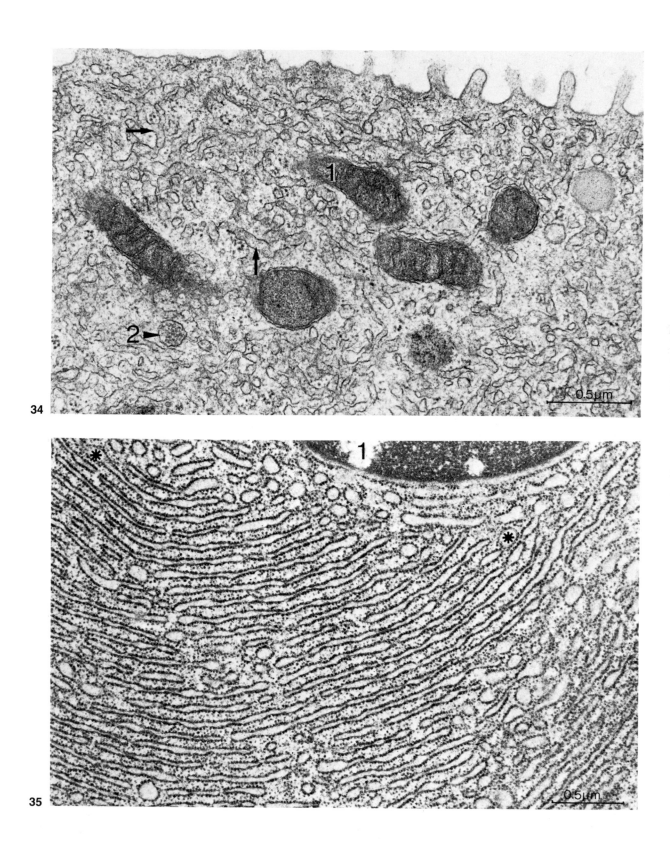

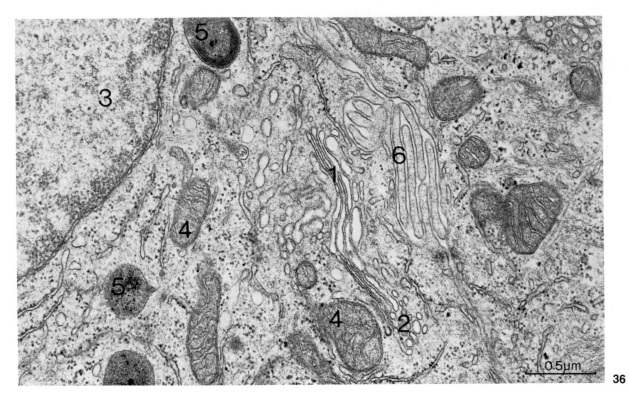

Fig. 36. Prominent **Golgi complex** in a salivary duct epithelial cell from the submandibular gland of a cat. This organelle consists of a low stack (dictyosome) of flattened saccules or cisternae (**1**), together with the adjacent vesicles and vacuoles (**2**) formed by budding off from the free edges of the cisternae (see also Fig. 23). **3** = Nucleus; **4** = Mitochondria; **5** = Lysosomes; **6** = Interdigitating processes of adjoining cells. Magnification 38,000×.

Fig. 37. A very elaborate **Golgi complex** consisting of at least ten individual stacks (**1**) (= dictyosomes) of sacculi which, however, might be interconnected with each other (from cultured human umbilical vein endothelial cell). Notice also numerous secondary lysosomes (**2**) close to the Golgi complex. Magnification 16,000×.

Fig. 38. This **Golgi complex** with its dictyosomes (**1**) and abundant vesicular components is arranged like the leaves of a flower around a centriole (**2**). Several of the vesicles display a fuzzy outer coat and an electron dense interior and represent coated vesicles (○). The dictyosomes appear to communicate along their outer and inner aspects (= forming and mature faces) with cisternae of the SER (∗). Because of this close topographical and possibly functional interrelationship between *G*olgi complex, *e*ndoplasmic *r*eticulum and, *l*ysosomes, the entire structure is called **GERL-complex** (from baboon mesenchymal cell of the cerebral dura mater). Magnification 30,000×.

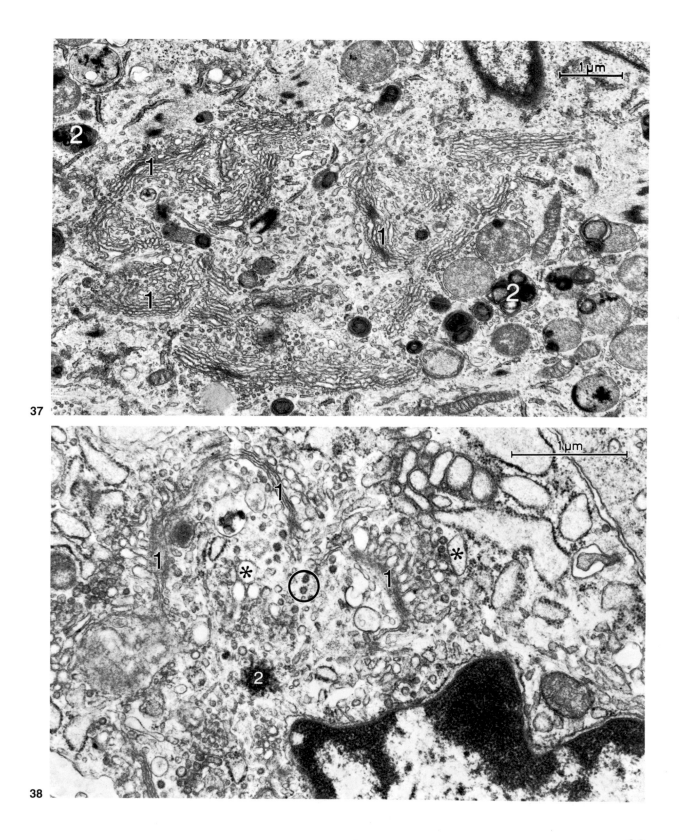

Nuclei of epithelial cells

Chromosomes

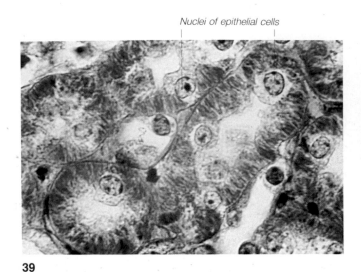

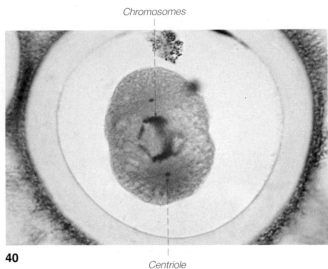

39

40

Centriole

Fig. 39. Light microscopic illustration of **mitochondria** with a special technique (according to Fernandez-Galiano) within the epithelial cells of kidney tubules (proximal convoluted tubules, for details see p. 171). The mitochondria appear as blackish filamentous structures aligned in parallel rows in the basal cytoplasm. Compare with the electron micrograph shown in Figure 28. Magnification 960×.

Fig. 40. Light micrograph of **centrioles** located at the poles of an oocyte undergoing meiotic divisions. From ovary of *Ascaris megalocephala sive equorum,* a large intestinal nematode parasite of horses. Iron hematoxylin staining. Magnification 960×.

Fig. 41. a) **Mitochondria** crowded together in a skeletal muscle fiber from the tongue of a cat. The variations in shape and size of the organelles are partly real and partly caused by the plane of the section. Several of the mitochondria contain dense granules (►) within their matrix which is subdivided by numerous narrow membrane bound electron lucent cavities, the cristae intramitochondriales. Because of these such mitochondria are classified as *crista-type* which is the most frequent representative of this organelle. Magnification 34,000×.

b) High-power view of a **mitochondrion** with well-developed and evenly spaced cristae aligned in parallel to each other but perpendicularly to the organelles' long axis. The cristae represent disk-like folds or pleats of the inner mitochondrial membrane and, in this case, they span almost the entire width of the mitochondrion. The arrowheads (►) indicate sites of continuity between the inner mitochondrial membrane with that of a crista (from cultured human endothelial cell). Magnification 58,000×.

c) Three elongated **mitochondria** from rat hepatocyte showing cristae which are oriented not only in parallel to each other but also to the organelles' long axis. Magnification 54,000×.

d) **Mitochondria** classified as "*tubular*" in type because their internal structure consists of tubules instead of cristae. Since the tubules are often twisted and curved (►) they usually appear as rounded or ovoid membrane profiles (from feline adrenal gland). Magnification 38,000×.

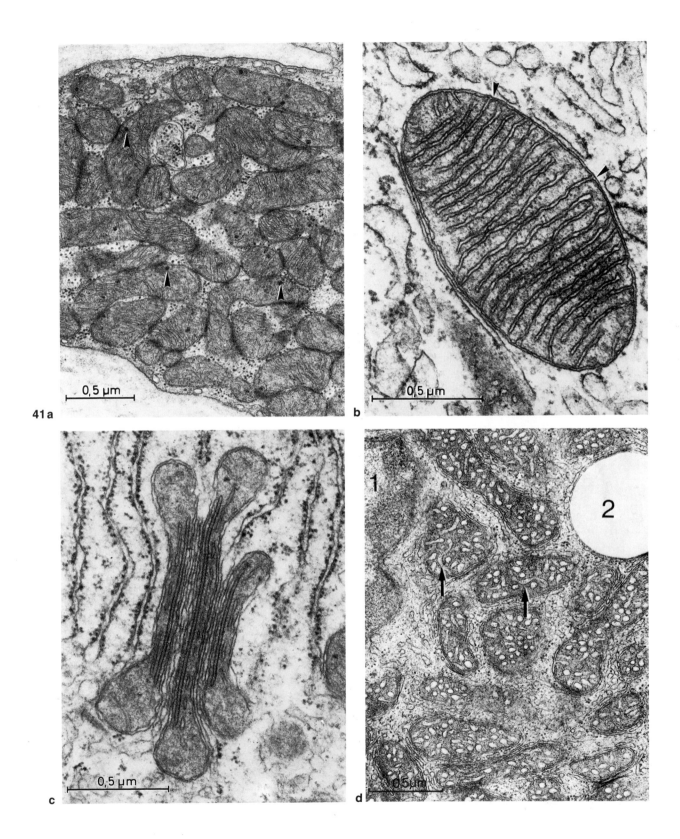

41a

b

c

0,5 µm

0,5 µm

0,5 µm

0,5µm

1

2

d

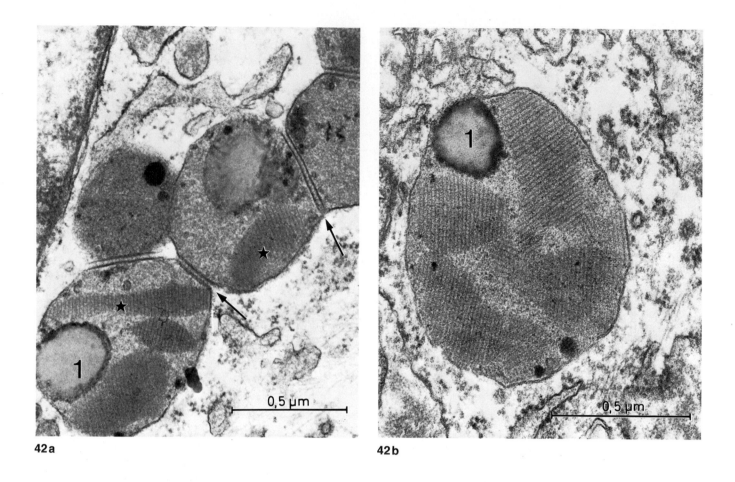

42 a

42 b

Fig. 42. Membrane-bound cytoplasmic corpuscles from human umbilical vein endothelial cells in situ displaying paracrystalline inclusions (★). When lying close together the adjoining membranes of these corpuscles are cross-connected in a zig-zag fashion by a delicate thread (→). Since these structures stain positively for acid phosphatase (not shown here) and usually reveal pleomorphic contents they are believed to represent a distinct group of **secondary lysosomes.**
b) In one of these organelles the interior is completely occupied by paracrystalline inclusions of varying configuration. **1** Lipid droplets. Magnifications 60,000× and 72,000×, respectively.

Fig. 43. **Peroxisomes (1)** in a rat hepatocyte show a finely granular homogeneous matrix together with an irregularly outlined electron dense inclusion known as the nucleoid (★), which is characteristic for this organelle in some species. **2** = Glycogen granules. Magnification 31,000×.

Fig. 44. Two distinct membrane-bound corpuscles (**1**) stuffed with vesicles represent typical **multivesicular bodies,** whereas two other similar globules (**2**) display fewer vesicles and a translucent interior. The latter two may represent multivesicular bodies undergoing degradation or forming (from baboon jugular vein endothelial cell). Magnification 44,000×.

Fig. 45. a) **Autophagic vacuole** in a rat liver cell. The vacuole contains profiles of SER (**1**) and an intact mitochondrion (**2**). After fusion with primary lysosomes, these vacuoles become "cytolysosomes" or "autolysosomes". Magnification 48,000×.
b) Large **secondary lysosomes** surrounded by ill-defined membranes. The globular contents consist of lipids (**1**), also seen lying free in the cytoplasm (1_1). These structures probably represent cytolysosomes converting to **residual bodies** (reticulum cell from rat thymus). Magnification 25,000×.

26

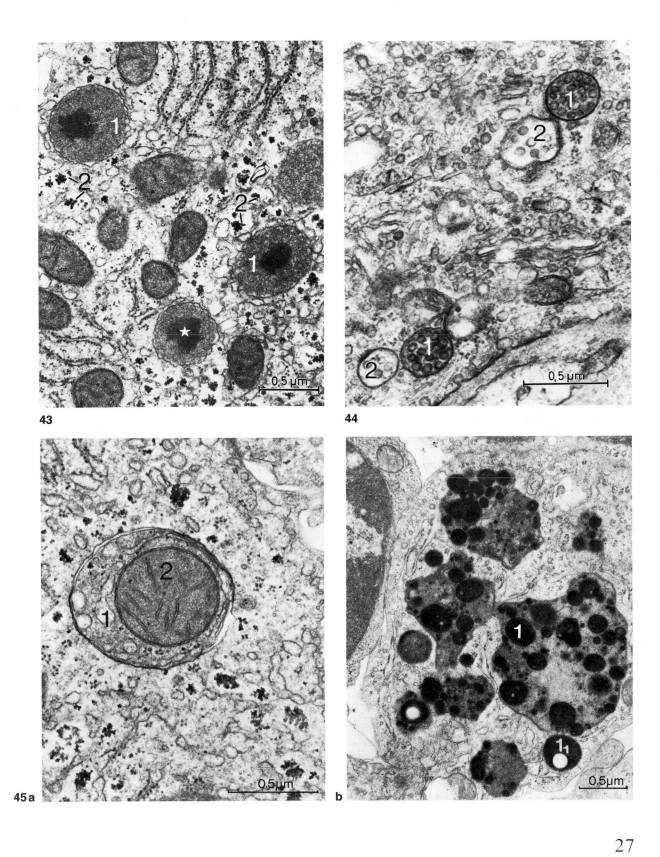

43

0,5 µm

44

0,5 µm

45 a

0,5 µm

b

0,5µm

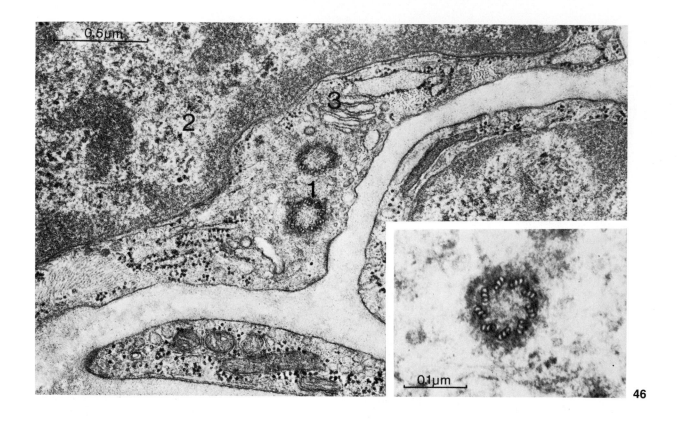

Fig. 46. Transverse and oblique sections of two **centrioles** (**1**) that together constitute the diplosome (fibroblast from feline connective tissue). Like most examples, neither of the two centrioles is cut exactly parallel or perpendicular to the long axis of the tubular units that constitute the wall of this organelle. Note that in this case, contrary to the rule, the long axes of the centrioles are not perpendicular to each other. **2** Nucleus; **3** Part of a Golgi dictyosome. The inset shows a centriole in perfect cross-section, displaying its "wall" composed of nine longitudinally oriented units, each of which consists of three microtubules joined together (= triplets). Magnification 50,000× and 160,000×.

Fig. 47. **Microtubules** (→) in longitudinal section converging upon a centriole (**1**) in rat thymocyte. The walls of these tubules (inner diameter: 6–10 nm, outer diameter: 20–26 nm) do not consist of a unit membrane but of 11–13 parallel filaments, each representing a chain of protein molecules known as tubulin. Magnification 69,000×.

Fig. 48. a) Small bundles (**1**) of fine parallel **filaments** (diameter 10 nm) in a rat intestinal epithelial cell. Magnification 56,000×.
b) Structurally similar filaments arranged in much coarser bundles (**1**) found in human epidermal cells. These bundles correspond to the tonofibrils seen by light microscopy (see Fig. 478). **2** Nucleus; **3** Melanin granule. Magnification 32,000×.

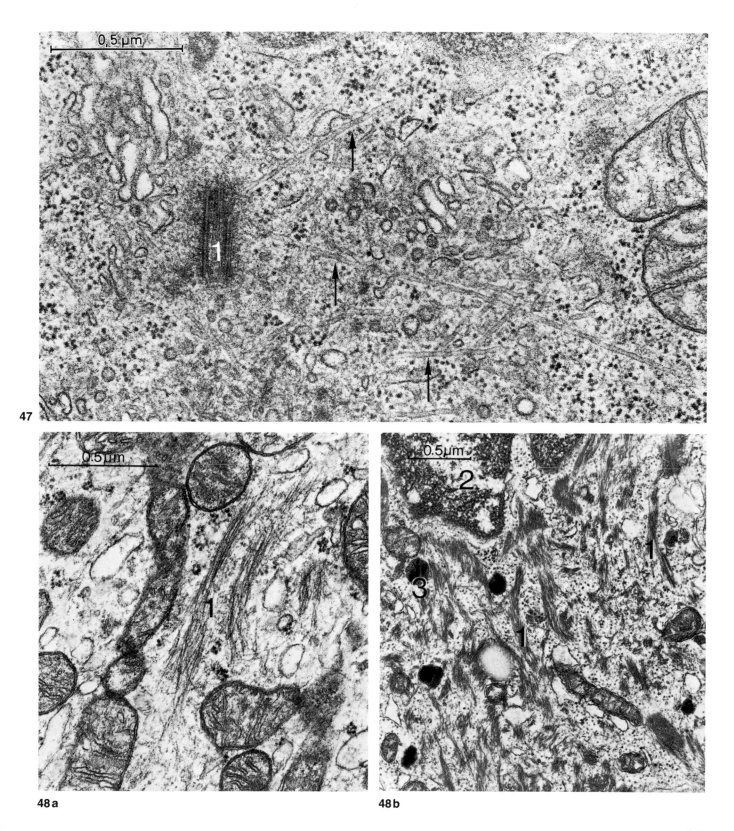

0.5 µm

47

0.5µm

1

48 a

0.5µm

2

3

1

1

48 b

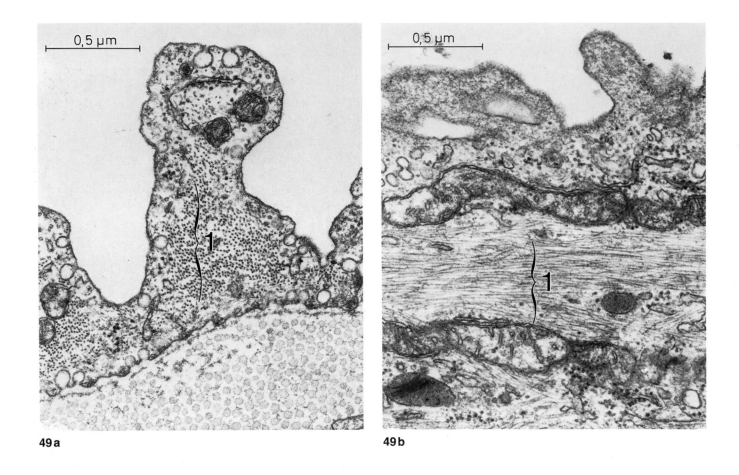

49a

49b

Fig. 49. **Intermediate or 10 nm filaments** (**1**) in cross- (**a**) and longitudinal section (**b**) within endothelial cells from rabbit venous valve (**a**) and baboon middle meningeal artery (**b**). This type of intracytoplasmic filament is mainly composed of the proteins desmin and vimentin and serves predominantly cytoskeletal functions, as exemplified in this case by an orientation strictly parallel to the blood stream. Magnification for (a) and (b) 49,000×.

Fig. 50. The two electron micrographs illustrate so-called **stress fibers** (**1**) in cross- (**a**) and longitudinal section (**b**) within endothelial cells lining the middle meningeal artery of a baboon. These fibers are bundles of parallel actin filaments (= microfilaments) with patches of myosin (= dense bodies) interspersed (►). This type of intracytoplasmic filaments provides tensile strength. Note also the close structural resemblance of stress fibers with the filament bundles (**2**) and their dense bodies (→) seen in the underlying smooth muscle cells. L = Vascular lumen. Magnification for (a) and (b) 55,000×.

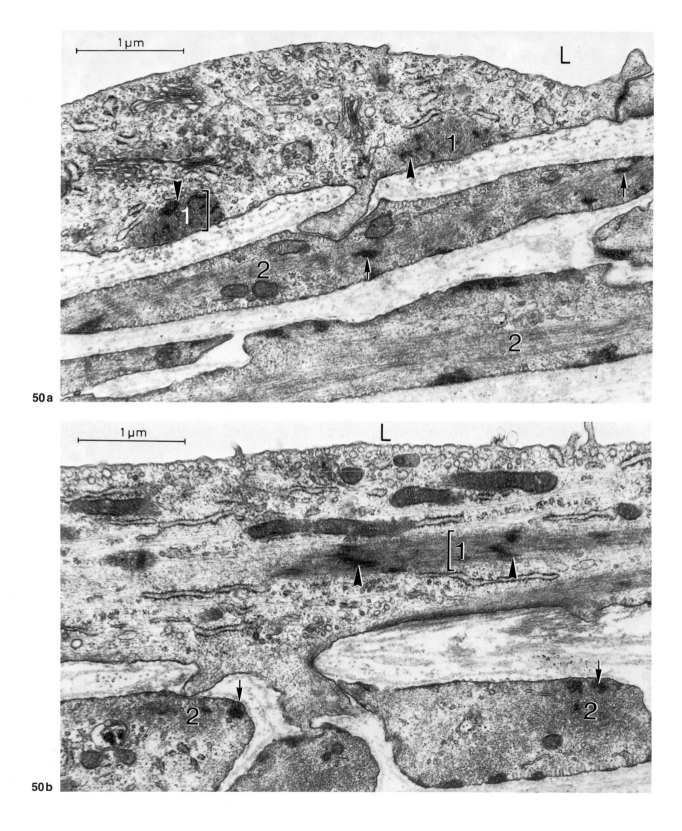

50a

50b

Cytology – Cell inclusions

Rod-shaped crystalloids in interstitial cells

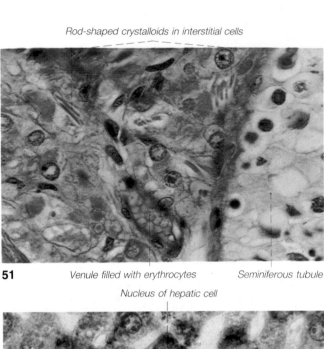

51   *Venule filled with erythrocytes*   *Seminiferous tubule*

Nucleus of a ganglion cell

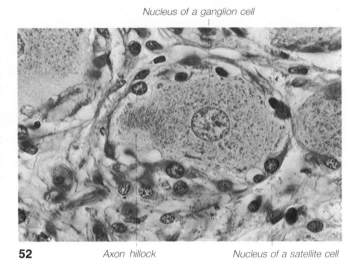

52   *Axon hillock*   *Nucleus of a satellite cell*

Nucleus of hepatic cell

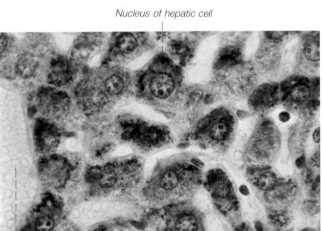

Central vein stuffed with erythrocytes   **53**

Secretion granules

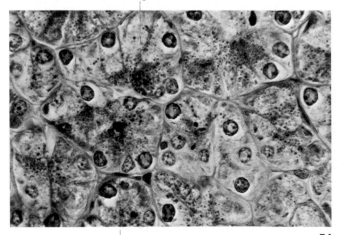

Lumen of serous acinus   **54**

Fig. 51. Part of a seminiferous tubule from human testis with adjacent interstitial (Leydig) cells that contain characteristic rod-shaped proteinaceous crystalloids known as the **crystals of Reinke.** Mallory-azan staining. Magnification 600×.

Fig. 52. Lipofuscin granules accumulated beside the axon hillock of a human spinal ganglion cell. This endogenous pigment is situated in residual bodies and represents the indigestible leftovers of lysosomal activity. It is sometimes known as "wear and tear" or "detrition" pigment. Mallory-azan staining. Magnification 600×.

Fig. 53. Rat liver cells selectively stained for **glycogen,** which appears as fine granules or coarser clumps colored magenta (courtesy of Prof. H. J. Clemens, Munich). PAS-hemalum staining. Magnification 600×.

Fig. 54. Serous acini (alveoli) of human submandibular gland with many red-stained **secretory granules** of various sizes showing different degrees of acidophilia. Mallory-azan staining. Magnification 600×.

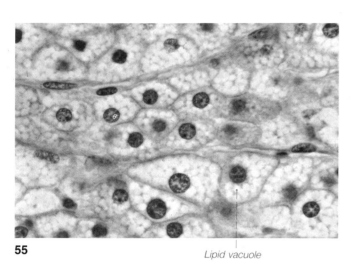

55

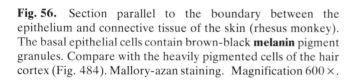
Lipid vacuole

Fig. 55. Clusters of polygonal cells filled with translucent **vacuoles** and thus referred to as "spongiocytes" (zona fasciculata of human adrenal gland). The vacuolation is due to the extraction of lipids by the organic solvents used in routine histological processing (see p. 1). Mallory-azan staining. Magnification 600×.

Fig. 56. Section parallel to the boundary between the epithelium and connective tissue of the skin (rhesus monkey). The basal epithelial cells contain brown-black **melanin** pigment granules. Compare with the heavily pigmented cells of the hair cortex (Fig. 484). Mallory-azan staining. Magnification 600×.

Fig. 57. Human lung alveoli containing siderophages or "heart failure cells" which develop in chronic pulmonary congestion by the progressive phagocytosis of the hematogenous pigment **hemosiderin.** Nuclear fast red staining. The iron is demonstrated by the Turnbull Prussian blue reaction, an important technique in histopathology. Magnification 600×.

Fig. 58. Section of a medullary sinus of a lymph node (human lung) containing numerous macrophages filled with dust particles, an **exogenous pigment.** This phenomenon is known as anthracosis (anthrax = coal). Mallory-azan staining. Magnification 380×.

Epithelial cells with melanin granules *Connective tissue*

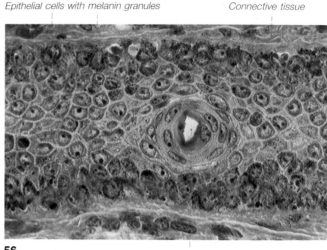

56 *Duct of a sweat gland*

Alveolar phagocytes filled with hemosiderin granules

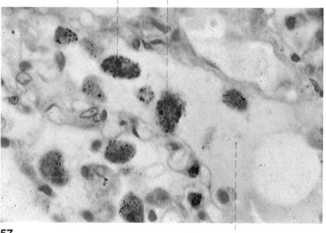

57 *Lumen of alveolus*

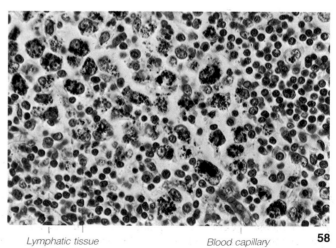

Lymphatic tissue *Blood capillary* **58**

33

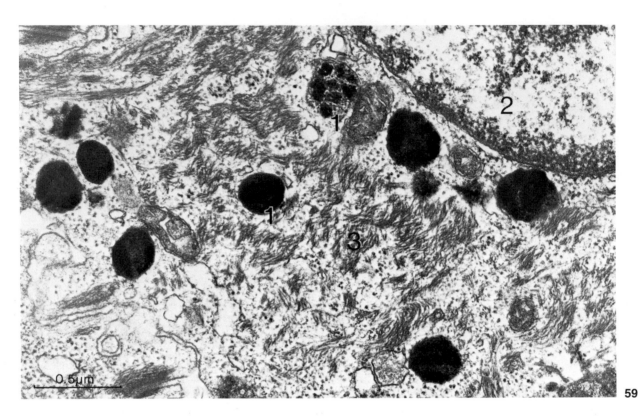

0.5 µm

59

Fig. 59. **Melanin granules** or melanosomes (**1**) in various stages of maturation in a human epidermal cell. **2** Nucleus; **3** Intracytoplasmic filaments. Magnification 45,000 ×.

Fig. 60. Membrane bound **secretory granules** (**1**) of various sizes in the apical portions of rat exocrine pancreatic cells. **2** Nucleus; **3** Lumen of acinus; **4** Mitochondria. Magnification 18,000 ×.

Fig. 61. a) **Lipid droplets** of various sizes. The limiting membranes are poorly defined because they have the same high electron density as the material they enclose (rat renal tubular cell). Magnification 17,500 ×.
b) **Glycogen particles** occurring individually as in this micrograph are referred to as "β-particles" (diameter 15–30 nm). Note the distinct matrix granules (►) in the mitochondria (human skeletal muscle fiber). Magnification 50,000 ×.

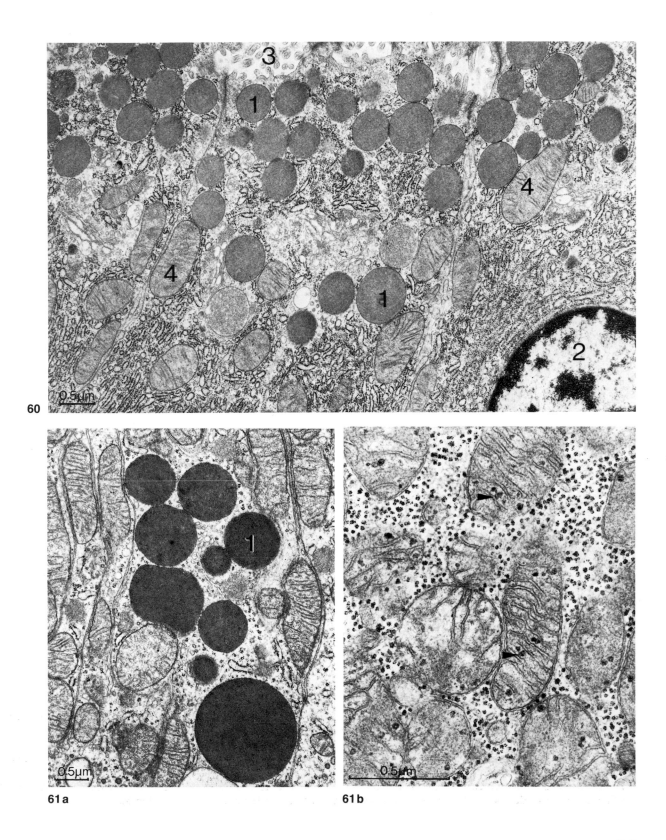

60

61a

61b

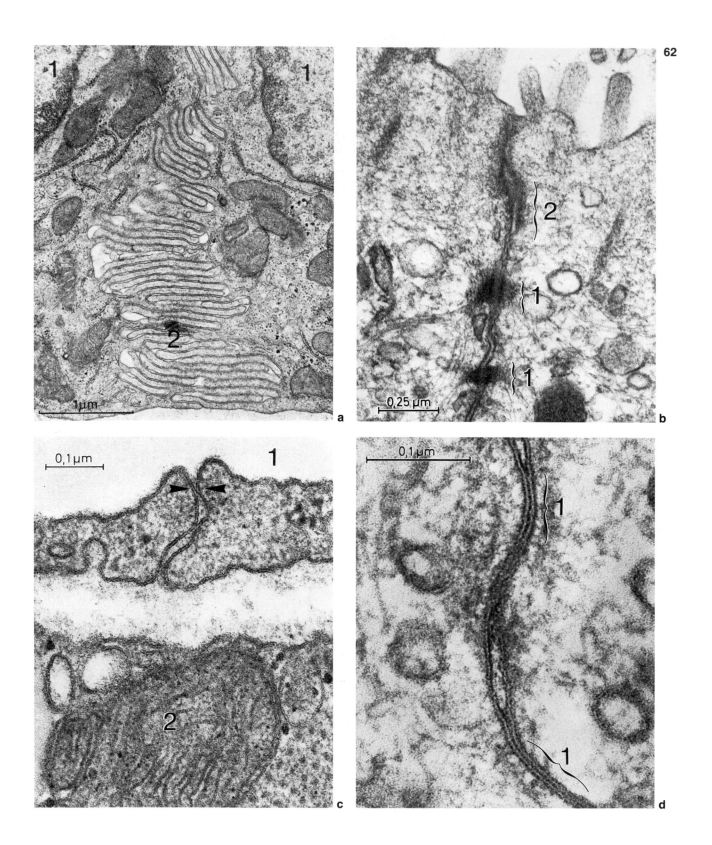

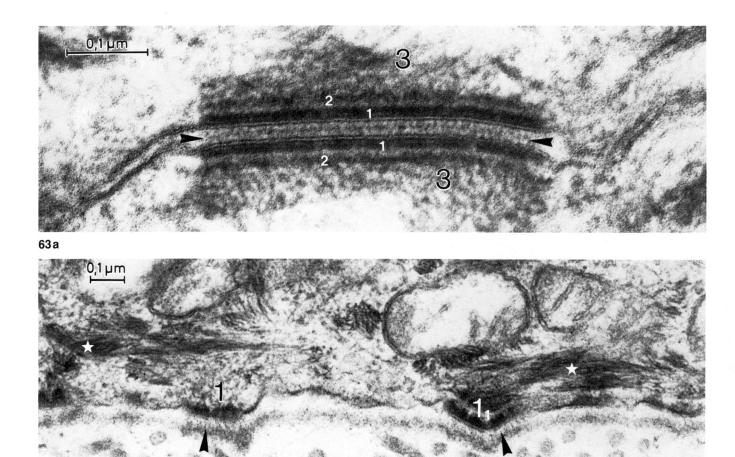

63a

63b

Fig. 63. a) Characteristic **desmosome** (= macula adherens) between epithelial cells of the epidermis from human skin. The trilaminar nature of the opposing plasmalemmata is clearly visible over the entire length of the desmosome the intercellular space of which is bisected by an electron dense line (►). Subjacent to the cytoplasmic face of the cell membranes lies an electron dense plaque (**1**) followed by a broader band of less electron opacity (**2**) into which tonofilaments (**3**) seem to enter and terminate. Magnification 205,000×.

b) Basal cell of human epidermis show **hemidesmosomes** (**1**), one of which (**1₁**) appears exactly as the halved desmosome illustrated in the preceding micrograph. Notice fine strands radiating from the hemidesmosomes' cell membrane (►) towards the opposing lamina densa of the underlying epithelial basal lamina. Note also tonofilaments (★) anchoring in the cytoplasmic condensations of the hemidesmosome. Magnification 85,000×.

Fig. 62. a) Numerous tightly interlacing cytoplasmic processes forming **interdigitations** that serve as a means of intercellular attachment between these two epithelials cells (salivary duct from feline submandibular gland). **1** Nuclei; **2** Desmosome. Magnification 24,000×.

b) **Junctional complex** between adjacent epithelial cells of guinea pig gallbladder. This type of attachment device corresponds to the terminal bar seen with the light microscope (see Fig. 88), but it reveals in this micrograph only two of its three components. Farthest down the intercellular space two desmosomes (**1**) (=macula adherens) can be seen followed by a zonula adherens (**2**), whereas the uppermost occluding zonule is obscured because it is sectioned tangentially. Magnification 62,000×.

c) Discrete spot-like fusion (► ◄) or **macula occludens** of the outer leaflets of opposing cell membranes in an interendothelial cleft of a cat myocardial capillary. **1** Capillary lumen; **2** Mitochondrion of cardiomyocyte. Magnification 145,000×.

d) Endothelial interface from rabbit thoracic aorta displaying fusion of the outer leaflets of the adjoining cell membranes over a longer distance (**1**) the **zonula occludens** (= tight junction). Magnification 270,000×.

37

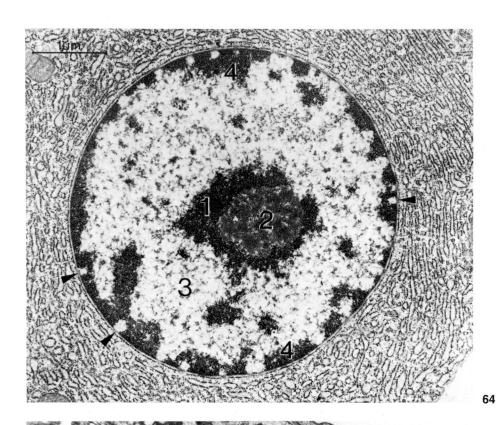

64

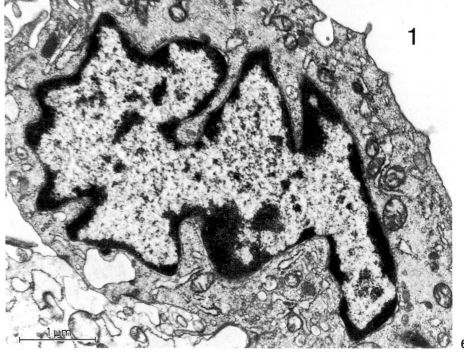

65

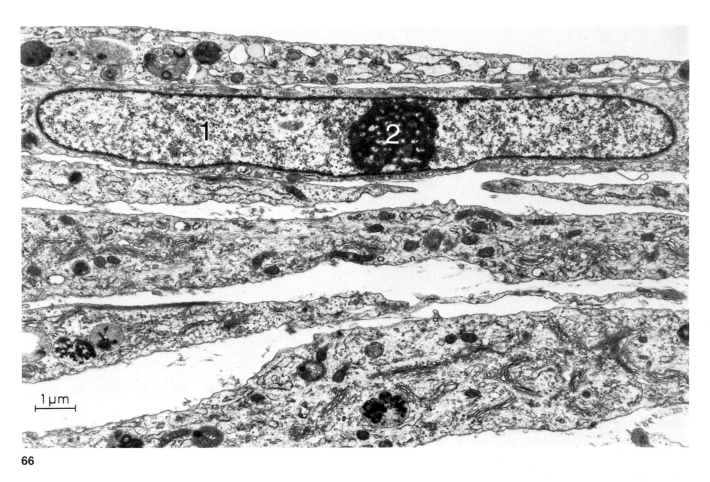

66

Fig. 66. Flat, elongated, **rod-shaped nucleus** of guinea pig endothelial cell grown in tissue culture for 7 days. When compared to figures 64 and 65 this nucleus contains almost no karyosomes (heterochromatin) but is nearly completely filled by euchromatin (**1**). In addition, the **nucleolus** (**2**) is large and prominent. Both these features indicate nuclear synthesis of RNA which is needed for protein synthesis in the cytoplasm. Use this micrograph to test your capacity in identifying the various cell components displayed in large numbers by these cultured cells. Magnification 10,000×.

Fig. 64. Typical **vesicular nucleus** from rat pancreatic acinar cell with smooth surface and **nucleolus** (**2**). The electron dense granular material represents condensed inactive **chromatin** (= heterochromatin) which occurs as nucleolus-associated **chromatin** (**1**) and often closely attached to the inner aspect of the nuclear envelope known here or elsewhere in the nuclear sap as karyosomes (**4**). The latter display several distinct circular lightenings (►) at the sites of the nuclear pores. The nuclear matrix or karyolymph (**3**) contains the uncoiled active euchromatin. The outer membrane of the nuclear envelope is clearly demarcated from its surrounding by its numerous attached ribosomes, the inner membrane is only poorly defined because of the closely applied chromatin. (More details of the nuclear envelope are shown in Figures 68–71). Magnification 19,000×.

Fig. 65. Intensely **indented nucleus** of an endothelial cell from human umbilical vein fixed by vascular perfusion under constant physiological pressure. The chromatin pattern is almost identical to that shown in the preceding micrograph but the nucleolus is not encountered in this section. **1** Vascular lumen. Magnification 20,000×.

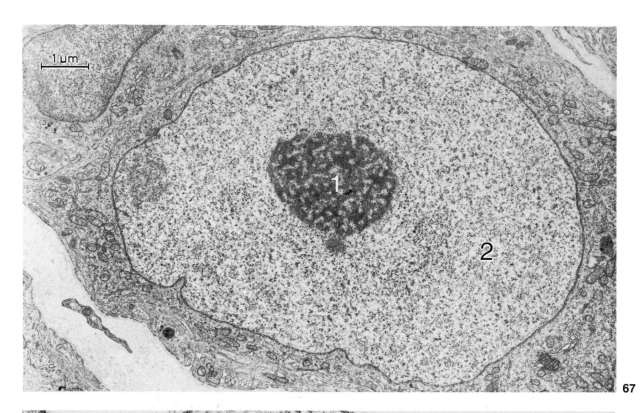

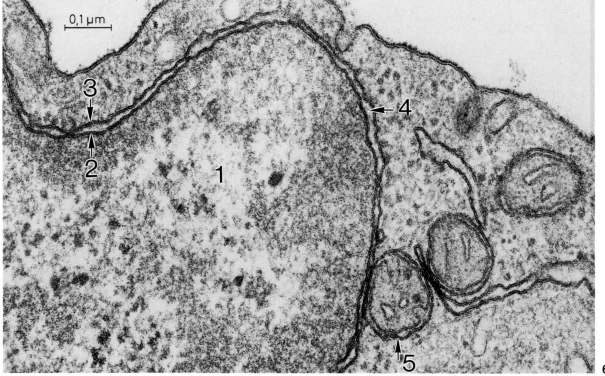

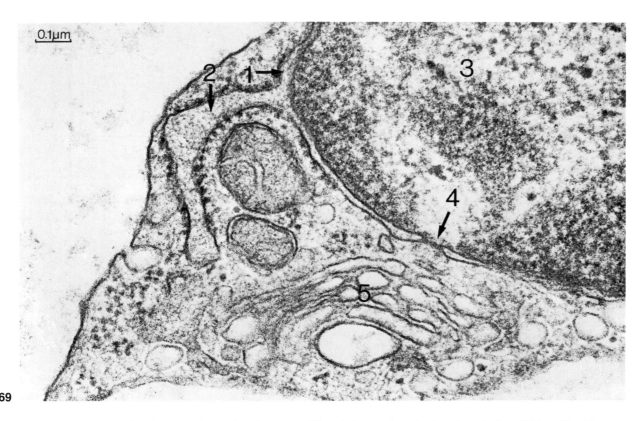

Fig. 69. Prominent communication between the **perinuclear space** (**1**) and the rough endoplasmic reticulum (**2**) in a fibroblast nucleus. **3** Nuclear matrix; **4** Nuclear pore; **5** Golgi saccules. Magnification 90,000×.

Fig. 67. Large smoothly contoured **nucleus** of a nerve cell from a minute autonomic ganglion found within a cat's pancreas. Note the prominent well-developed **nucleolus** (**1**) clearly revealing its coiled **nucleolonema** and the complete replacement of heterochromatin by the uncoiled active euchromatin. The inner membrane of the nuclear envelope is also distinct due to the lack of adjacent chromatin particles. Magnification 12,000×.

Fig. 68. Part of an endothelial nucleus (**1**) clearly demonstrating the trilaminar nature of both its inner (**2**) and outer (**3**) membranes, which together with the perinuclear space (**4**) constitute the **nuclear envelope.** Note that the three-layered structure of the inner and outer mitochondrial membranes (**5**) is also apparent. Magnification 120,000×.

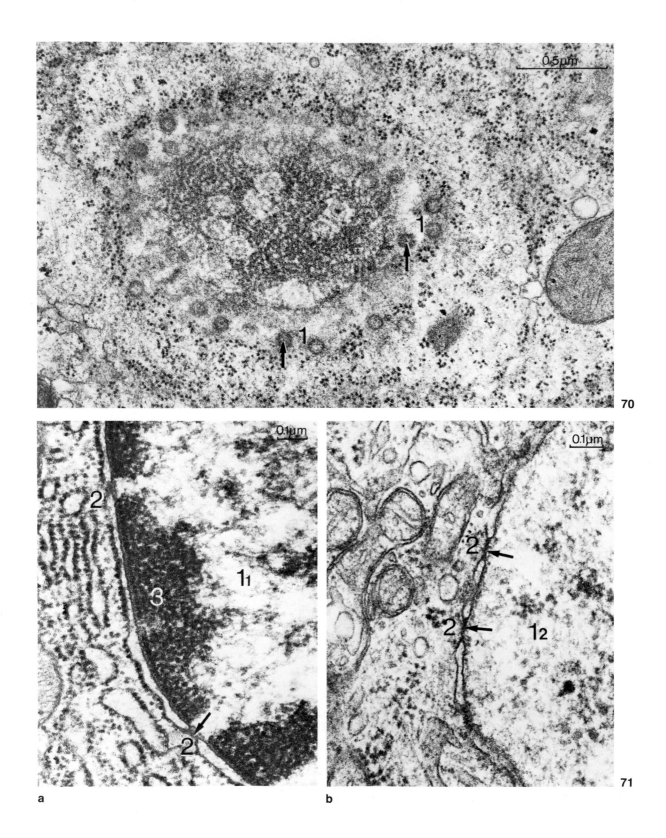

a

b

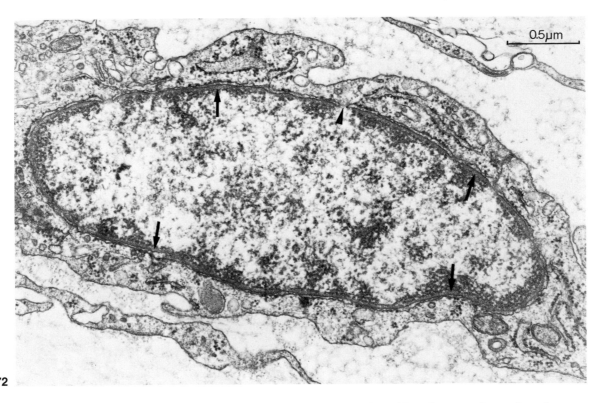

72

Fig. 72.   Prominent **fibrous lamina** (→) in a fibroblast nucleus (subcutaneous tissue, rat) positioned as a continuous layer between the inner nuclear membrane and the chromatin. Only at the sites of the nuclear pores (►) does the lamina fibrosa reveal corresponding circular disruptions. Magnification 38,000×.

Fig. 70.   Tangential view of a rat liver cell **nucleus** showing numerous **pores** (1). These appear as circular openings (inner diameter 35 nm) in routine electron micrographs and show a central knob-like condensation (→) in appropriate sections. The pores are potential avenues of communication between nucleoplasm and cytoplasm and are often referred to as a "pore complex" because of their intricate substructure (not seen in this micrograph). Magnification 48,000×.

Fig. 71. a), b)   Parts of nuclei from an exocrine pancreatic cell (1₁) and a ganglion cell (1₂) of the rat. The inner and outer nuclear membranes are continuous with each other round the periphery of the distinct **pores** (2), thereby sealing the perinuclear space. In addition, the pores are often bridged by a delicate "membrane", the diaphragm. Immediately subjacent to the inner surface of the nuclear envelope of some cell types (Figs. 71a, 72) is a fine filamentous layer, the lamina fibrosa. **3** Chromatin. Magnification 78,000× and 86,000×.

Light microscopy – Sex chromatin and mitosis

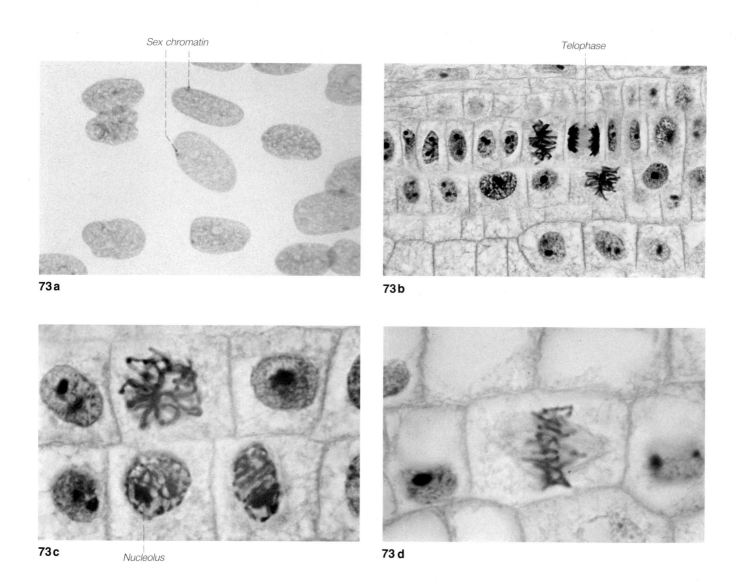

Sex chromatin

Telophase

73a

73b

Nucleolus

73c

73d

Fig. 73. a) **Sex chromatin** corresponds to one of the two X-chromosomes of females that remains condensed (inactive) in the interphase nucleus and therefore, represents heterochromatin. To demonstrate this special chromatin particle or **Barr body** a smear of the buccal mucosa is prepared and stained specifically for DNA as, e.g., with either thionin or leuco-fuchsin. The sex chromatin is visible in this case as a faintly staining granule immediately adjacent to the nuclear envelope. Thionin staining. Magnification 960×.
b–h) Different stages of **karyokinesis** from mitotic cell divisions, whose final stage, the division of the cytoplasm (cytokinesis) which results in two separate daughter cells, is not shown. To demonstrate cell divisions histologically, rapidly growing tissues with a high mitotic rate such as cell cultures, embryos or, as in this case, germinating plant seedlings are used.
b) Low-power micrograph from the tip of the root of a bean seedling *(Vicia faba)* showing many closely apposed cells whose nuclei exhibit different stages of karyokinesis. At the right side of the upper row of cells are two cells each of which is exactly half the size of the parent cell and which therefore represent the daughter cells resulting from a complete mitosis. In the center of the upper row are an early telophase (see also Fig. 73h) and a late metaphase (see also Fig. 73e). Iron hematoxylin staining. Magnification 500×.
c) At the lower margin of this micrograph two nuclear divisions showing early stages of **prophase** with distinct nucleoli are visible. Above these cells a **metaphase** in polar view can be seen giving the appearance of a **monaster**.

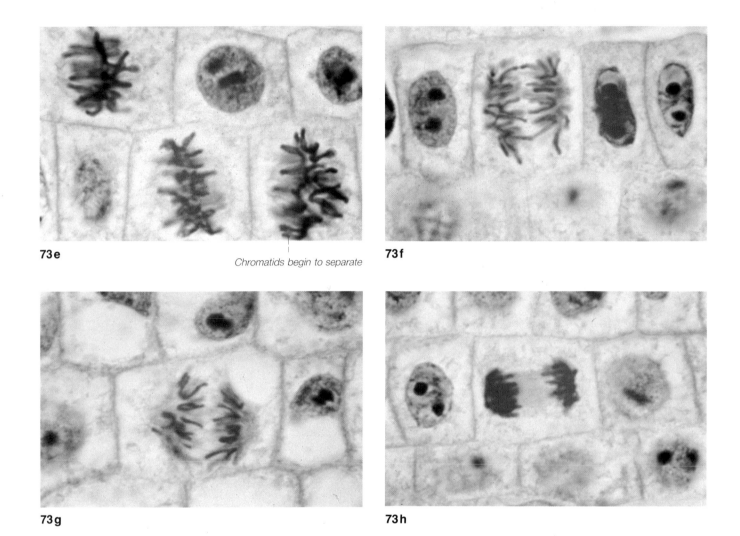

73e

Chromatids begin to separate

73f

73g

73h

d) **Metaphase** in lateral view with the chromosomes situated midway in the spindle and aligned in the equatorial plate. The prominent mitotic spindle consists of fibers that correspond to bundles of microtubules, which connect the kinetochore of each of the chromosomes with the opposite poles of the spindle apparatus. The centrioles are located at these sites in animal cells. Since cells of higher plants lack this organelle, the reader is kindly referred to Figure 40.

e) Late **metaphases** in oblique section so that the precise orientation of the chromosomes is not completely obvious. At certain points, particularly of the lower right metaphase, sister chromatids, originating from each chromosome by reduplication in the S-phase and destined to become the definitive chromosomes of the two future daughter cells, begin to separate.

f) Early **anaphase** with all sister chromatids separated into daughter chromatids that have been pulled apart and moved toward the poles.

g) Later stage of **anaphase** displaying discrete interpolar spindle fibers which course parallel to each other and in the direction of the axis between the poles (in animal cells between the centrioles located at the poles).

h) Early **telophase** with an increasing clumping of chromosomes into a homogeneous, intensely staining basophilic mass. The continuous spindle fibers are still clearly visible.

Figs. 73c–h: Iron hematoxylin staining. Magnification 1,250×.

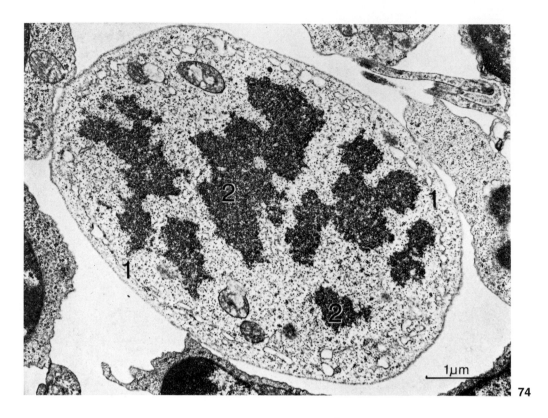

74

Fig. 74.   Low power electron micrograph of **prophase** in a rat thymocyte. The condensing chromosomes (**2**) are still surrounded by remnants of the nuclear envelope (**1**).   Magnification 16,000 ×.

Fig. 75.   Low power electron micrograph of **metaphase** in mesenchymal cell of chick chorioallantoic membrane. Remnants of the nuclear envelope may be observed at arrow heads.   **1** Chromosomes. Magnification 14,000 ×.

Fig. 76.   **Anaphase** in an endothelial cell lining embryonic vessels of chick chorioallantoic membrane.   **1** Chromosomes. Magnification 14,000 ×.

In both figures neither centrioles nor the microtubular mitotic spindle are included in the respective section.

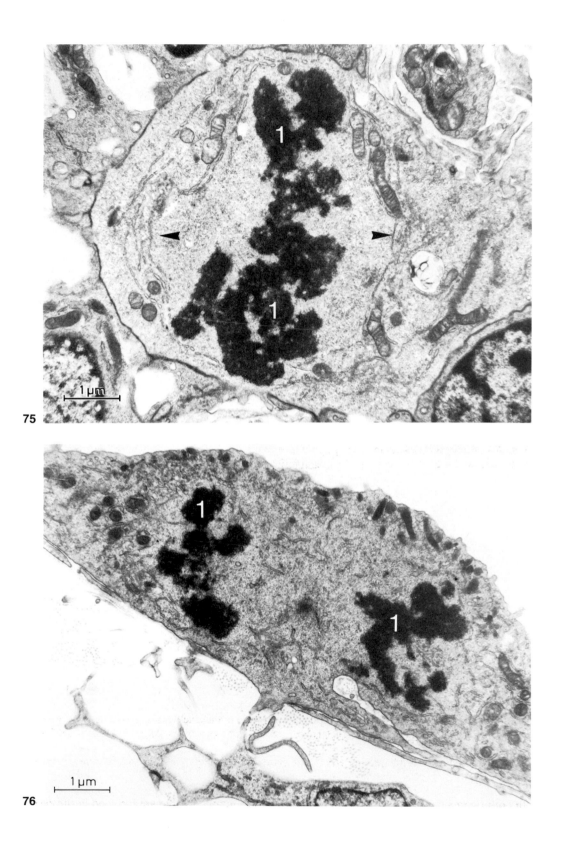

75

76

Histology

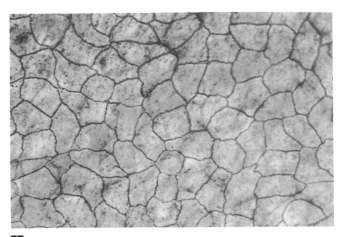

77

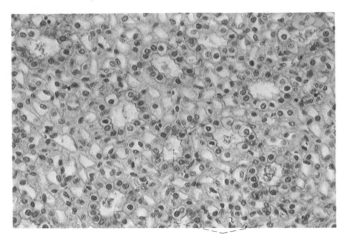

78 *Lumina of collecting tubule*

Goblet cell

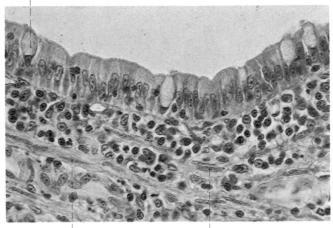

79 *Smooth muscle cells in the lamina propria*

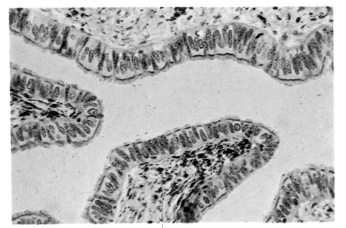

80 *Connective tissue in fold of mucous membrane*

Fig. 77. *En face* view of a thin spread of a cat peritoneum treated with silver nitrate. The cells of this simple squamous epithelium are clearly outlined by silver deposits at the cellular interfaces. The nuclei have not been counterstained. Magnification 240×.

Fig. 78. Simple cuboidal epithelium lining collecting tubules in the renal medulla (rabbit). Thyroid follicles are also commonly used to demonstrate this type of epithelium (see Fig. 460). Mallory-azan staining. Magnification 240×.

Fig. 79. Simple columnar epithelium from the cat jejunum showing several goblet cells (unicellular glands). The striated border at the luminal surface of the absorptive epithelial cells is better seen at higher magnification (Fig. 91). Note smooth muscle cells in the lamina propria. H & E staining. Magnification 380×.

Fig. 80. Simple ciliated columnar epithelium lining the mucosal folds of the human uterine (fallopian) tube. Higher magnification would show that the narrow black line at the base of the cilia consists of many tiny dots corresponding to the basal bodies (cf. Figs. 87, 92, 97). Iron hematoxylin staining. Magnification 240×.

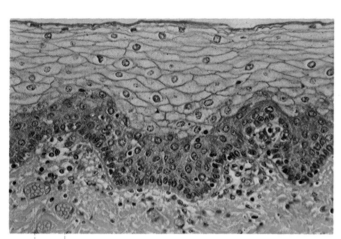

Venules stuffed with erythrocytes   **81**

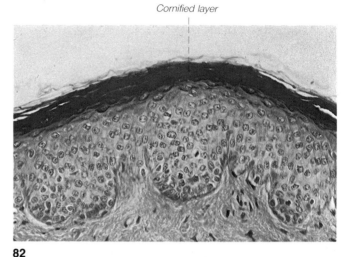

Cornified layer

82

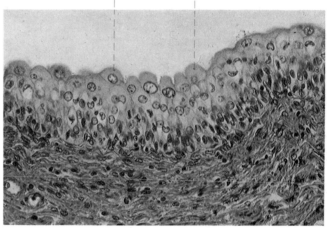

Surface cells with superficial layer of condensed cytoplasm

83

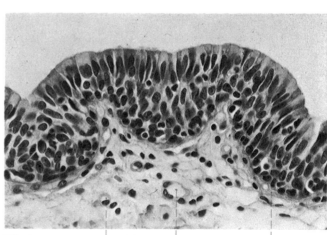

84   Small blood vessels within lamina propria   Basement membrane

Fig. 81. Human vaginal epithelium, an example of the non-keratinizing variety of stratified squamous epithelia. All of the cells contain nuclei. The classification of stratified epithelium is always based on the shape of the cells in the uppermost layer. As can be seen here, only the cells in this layer have the characteristic squamous shape. Goldner staining. Magnification 240×.

Fig. 82. Slightly keratinized stratified squamous epithelium from the skin of human nostrils (cf. Fig. 481). The surface cells are non-nucleated and have become completely transformed into horny plates, forming the cornified layer. Mallory-azan staining. Magnification 240×.

Fig. 83. Transitional epithelium from human urinary bladder. The appearance of this epithelium varies greatly depending on the state of contraction or distention of the hollow organs which it lines. In routine histologic specimens it usually appears as "stratified" and the student should thus consider transitional epithelium when dealing with stratified epithelia in general. Characteristic features of transitional epithelium are the surface cells, often binucleate with a superficial zone of condensed darker staining cytoplasm (see also Fig. 90). Since this epithelium is the typical lining of the excretory passages of the urinary system (from renal calyces to urethra) it has recently been named "urothelium" or "urothel". Mallory-azan-staining. Magnification 240×.

Fig. 84. True stratified columnar epithelium from human female urethra. This type of epithelium is very rare. In this case it has to be classified as columnar because the cells of its uppermost layer are columnar in appearance though all the other cells are not. Mallory-azan staining. Magnification 380×.

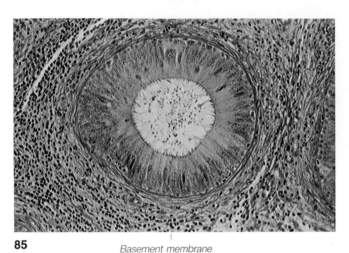

85

Basement membrane

Fig. 85. Pseudostratified columnar epithelium with stereocilia (human ductus epididymidis). This epithelium is classified as "pseudostratified" because all of its cells rest on the basement membrane, although not all of them reach the free surface. These details are usually invisible in ordinary histologic specimen due to thickness of section (see however, Fig. 87), but experience will teach the student that what might appear at first sight to be a "stratified" columnar epithelium is in most cases in fact pseudostratified and particularly so if equipped with either stereo- or motile cilia. In contrast to motile cilia, stereocilia lack basal bodies and their free ends are stuck together (see also Fig. 93). When viewed by electron microscopy (cf. Fig. 95), stereocilia are seen to be long branching cell processes lacking the characteristic structure of true motile cilia. Iron hematoxylin and benzo light Bordeaux staining. Magnification 150×.

Goblet cells

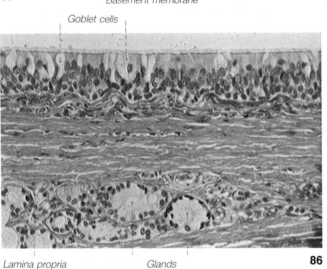

Lamina propria   *Glands*   **86**

Fig. 86. Ciliated pseudostratified columnar epithelium containing many goblet cells (human trachea). Since this type of epithelium occurs only in the respiratory tract, it is often called "respiratory epithelium". Mallory-azan staining. Magnification 240×.

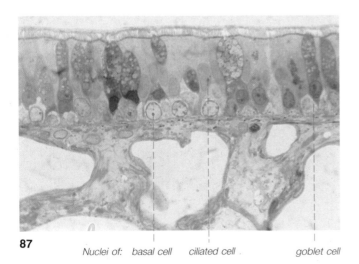

87

Nuclei of: basal cell   ciliated cell   goblet cell

Fig. 87. Plastic semi-thin section (thickness approx. 1 μm) of respiratory epithelium from rabbit nasal mucosa illustrates structural details to a better advantage. At least three rows of nuclei oriented parallel to each other and to the cell surface can be distinguished by means of their distinctly different chromatin pattern. Basal row: large poorly stained nuclei; middle row: prominently stained nuclei of the goblet cells; upper row: faintly but homogeneously colored ovoid nuclei of the ciliated cells displaying almost no chromatin. Compare this figure with the corresponding electron micrograph taken from same material and shown in Figure 97. Methylene blue-azure II staining. Magnification 380×.

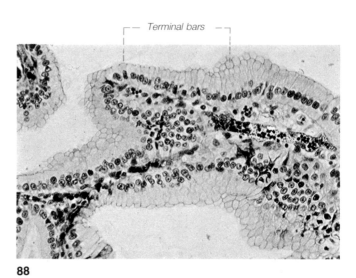

Terminal bars

88

Fig. 88. Mucosal fold covered by a tall simple columnar epithelium (human gallbladder). Where the epithelium is sectioned tangentially, a hexagonal array of blackish lines surrounds the apical parts of the cells. These lines are the "terminal bars" which electron microscopy shows to be a sequence of three different attachment devices forming a junctional complex (see Fig. 62b). Iron hematoxylin staining. Magnification 240×.

Vein filled with red blood cells

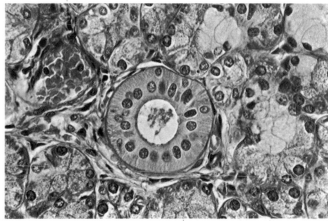

89   *Serous and mucous alveolus*

Fig. 89. Striated (salivary) duct from human submandibular gland. The basal portions of the columnar cells have a striated appearance because their mitochondria are oriented perpendicularly to the base of the cell. The electron microscopic equivalent of this basal striation is the "basal labyrinth" shown in Figure 28. This is a particularly well-differentiated Mallory-azan stain as can be seen from the orange-yellow color of the erythrocytes (cf. Fig. 12). Mallory-azan staining. Magnification 380×.

Binucleated surface cell   Crusta

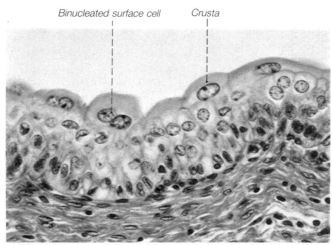

90

Fig. 90. Transitional epithelium from human urinary bladder. A specialization unique to this epithelium is the occurrence of a zone of condensed darker-staining cyptoplasm adjacent to the luminal surface. This zone contains a mixture of different glycoproteins. Electron microscopy reveals many filaments and membrane-bound oblong vacuoles in this region. Mallory-azan staining. Magnification 380×.

Basement membrane

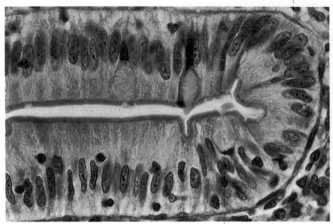

91

Goblet cell with nucleus

The three most common specializations found at epithelial surfaces are represented by cell processes of different shape and structure.

Fig. 91. Human intestinal epithelium illustrating the striated or brush border (stained a pale greyish violet), which is particularly well developed in all types of absorptive cells. Electron micrographs show it to be composed of numerous regularly arranged microvilli of uniform height (see Figs. 26, 27, 94). Mallory-azan staining. Magnification 600×.

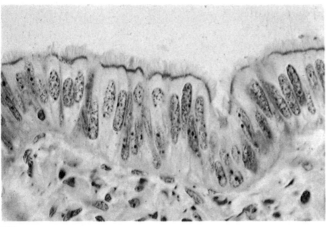

92

Fig. 92. The simple columnar epithelium of the human uterine (fallopian) tube possesses motile cilia (kinocilia) at its surface. These can easily be distinguished from either striated border or stereocilia by means of their basal bodies, here shown as a narrow bluish-black line. Although cilia are often overlooked because of their poor staining properties, they become clearly visible by refraction when the iris diaphragm of the microscope condenser is closed. Iron hematoxylin staining. Magnification 600×.

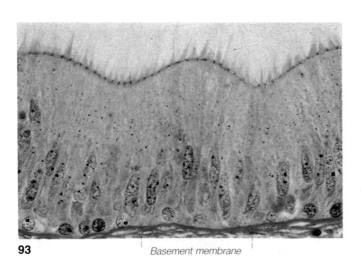

93

Basement membrane

Fig. 93. Photomicrograph of human ductus epididymidis. The nonmotile stereocilia of each cell surface are stuck together at their free ends and lack basal bodies. Electron micrographs show that they are unusually long branching cell processes (cf. Fig. 95). The extremely fine dark dots located between the apical ends of the epithelial cells correspond to cross sections of the terminal bars (see also Fig. 88). Hematoxylin and benzo light Bordeaux staining. Magnification 600×.

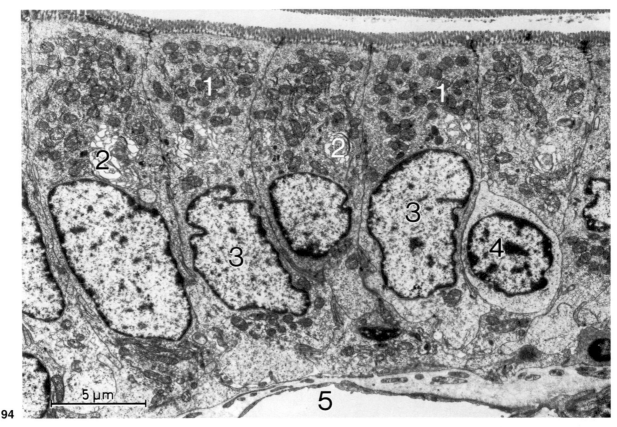

94

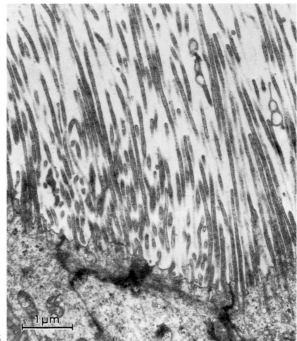

95

Fig. 94. Simple columnar epithelium from rat duodenum equipped with closely and regularly spaced microvilli of uniform size and shape (cf. Fig. 27). The supranuclear cyptoplasm of these cells is crowded with mitochondria (**1**) and it has dilated Golgi sacculi (**2**). **3** Nuclei of epithelial cells; **4** Nucleus of lymphoid cell migrating through the epithelium; **5** Lumen of fenestrated capillary. Magnification 5,000 ×.

Fig. 95. Stereocilia (from rat ductus deferens) represent another stable specialization of epithelial cell surfaces. These nonmotile cytoplasmic processes are composed, at the level of electron microscopy, of an abundance of extremely long microvilli. Magnification 13,000 ×.

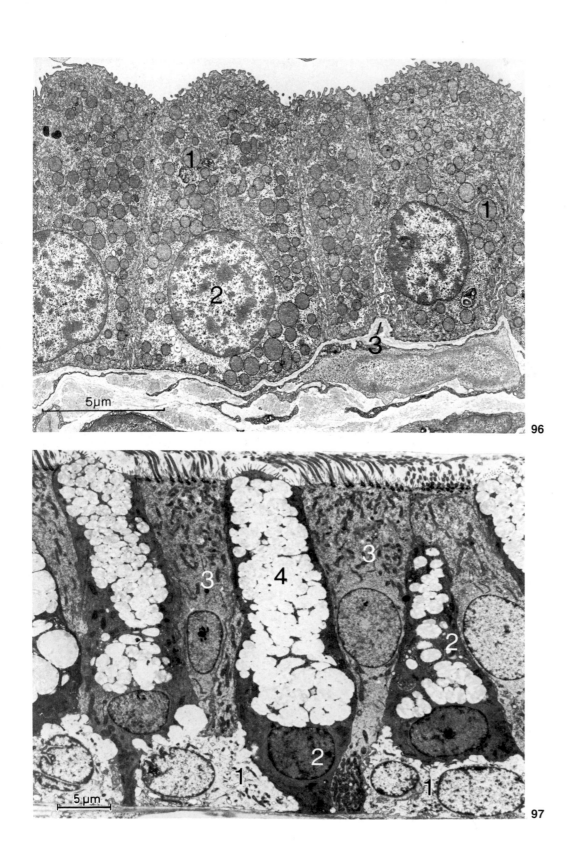

5µm

96

5µm

97

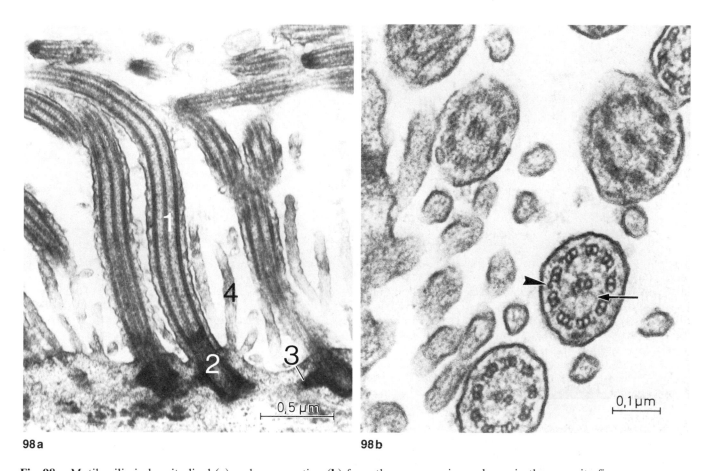

98a   98b

Fig. 98. Motile cilia in longitudinal (**a**) and cross-section (**b**) from the same specimen shown in the opposite figure.

a) One of the cilia (**1**) is cut mid-sagittaly and clearly reveals the central and two of its outer fibrils which actually consist of paired microtubules. The central pair terminates at the basal body (**2**), a modified centriole, whereas the outer fibrils are continuous with two of the microtubules constituting the triplets of the centrioles' wall. Faintly cross-striated rootlets (**3**) project from the basal bodies at right angles and appear as electron dense triangles. Note also the irregular microvilli (**4**) interspersed with the cilia. Magnification 39,000 ×.

b) Tranverse section through motile cilia disclose the trilaminar nature of their outer membrane and their complex internal structure. The latter consist of two single microtubules in the center of the axoneme encircled by nine uniformly spaced groups of paired microtubules (doublets); and hence this arrangement, universal in all kinocilia, is often referred to as the "9 + 2" structure. The central tubules are connected with the doublets by fine radiating condensations (→) whereas free "arms" (►) project from each doublet toward its counterclockwise neighbor. Magnification 120,000 ×.

Fig. 96. Simple low columnar epithelium from a respiratory bronchiole (cat). The cell surfaces show irregular short microvilli. The cytoplasm is uniformly filled with secretion granules (**1**) but the other details of its fine structure, such as the well-developed smooth ER, are not seen at this magnification. **2** Nucleus; **3** Basal lamina. Magnification 6,500 ×.

Fig. 97. Electron micrograph of pseudostratified ciliated columnar epithelium from rabbit nasal septum. All the cells rest upon the basement membrane but not all reach the surface. Three types of cells: (**1**) basal-, (**2**) goblet-, and (**3**) ciliated cells are clearly distinguishable, the nuclei of which are arranged in rows parallel to each other and to the surface. Note that between the cilia, readily identifiable by their electron dense basal bodies, numerous irregular microvilli project from the free surface of the same epithelial cell (for details see Fig. 98). **4** Dissolved mucous secretion. Magnification 2,700 ×.

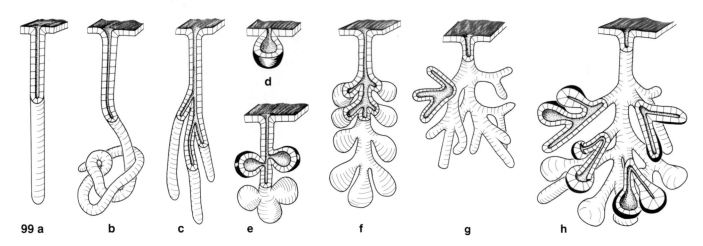

99 a   b   c   e   f   g   h

Fig. 99. The classification of exocrine glands is based on the shapes of their secretory units and the arrangement of their duct system.

a) Simple tubular gland with each secretory unit opening directly onto the epithelial surface, e.g., colonic crypts. **b)** Simple coiled tubular gland, e.g., skin sweat glands. **c)** Simple branched tubular gland with several secretory units emptying into a single unbranched secretory duct, e.g., gastric pyloric glands. **d)** Simple alveolar gland. **e)** and **f)** Simple branched alveolar glands, e.g., skin sebaceous glands. **g)** Compound tubular gland with the tubular secretory units leading into an elaborately branched duct system. Alveolar or acinar glands also have a compound duct system. **h)** Tubular and alveolar/acinar secretory units in the same gland. The different secretory portions can either follow one another in successive parts of the gland to form a "mixed tubuloalveolar or tubuloacinar" gland, e.g., sublingual and submandibular gland, or remain separate and unconnected as a "tubuloalveolar or tubuloacinar" gland. **g)** and **h)** are examples of compound glands, i.e., glands with a branched duct system.
See Table 5 for the classification of exocrine glands.

Nucleus of a goblet cell

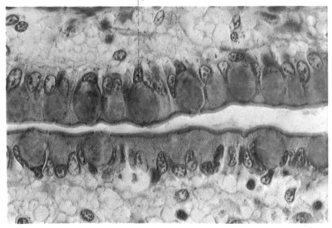

100

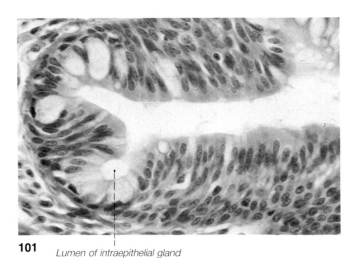

101   Lumen of intraepithelial gland

Fig. 100. Goblet cells in the epithelial lining of the ileum as examples of unicellular intraepithelial glands. With Mallory-azan staining all mucous secretory granules are brillant blue. Note the wedge-shaped nucleus in the "stem" of the goblet and the prominent striated border of the absorptive epithelium. Mallory-azan staining. Magnification 600×.

Fig. 101. Multicellular intraepithelial gland in the mucosa of the human nasal septum. Iron hematoxylin and benzo purpurin staining. Magnification 380×.

Lumen of epithelial crypt

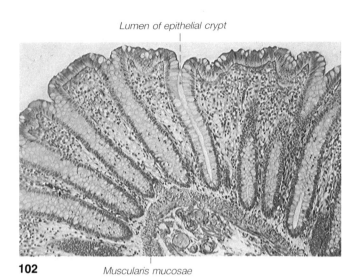

Lumina of two serous acini

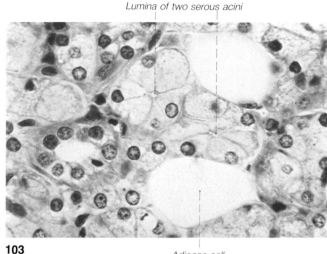

102   *Muscularis mucosae*

103   *Adipose cell*

Myoepithelial cells

Fig. 102. The crypts of the colonic mucosa (man) are the classic example of simple tubular glands. The crypt walls are composed mainly of secretory (goblet) cells. Since the crypts are not oriented exactly perpendicularly to the surface, they are often cut tangentially so that only parts lie in the plane of the section. Note the cross-sectioned smooth muscle of the muscularis mucosae at the base of the crypts. Mallory-azan staining. Magnification 95×.

Fig. 103. A transverse section of an acinar secretory unit is clearly visible in the upper central part of this micrograph (human parotid gland). Note the globular nuclei of the wedge-shaped secretory cells that border on a narrow lumen, the latter more obvious than usual (cf. Fig. 111). Mallory-azan staining. Magnification 600×.

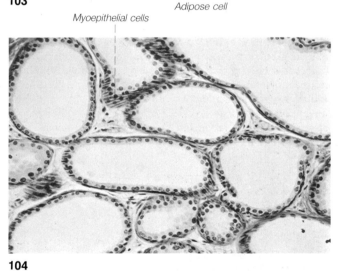

104

Cytoplasmic domes with secretory product

Fig. 104. Extremely wide lumina of alveolar secretory units of the ceruminous glands in human external auditory canal. Because of their apocrine secretory mechanism, they are commonly though misleadingly called large apocrine "sweat" glands. Mallory-azan staining. Magnification 150×.

Fig. 105. Single alveolar secretory unit from human apocrine sweat gland of axillary skin. The structural correlate of the apocrine secretion mechanism is represented by the domed apical portions of the glandular epithelial cells. This darker staining cytoplasm also contains the secretory product together with which it is pinched off into the glandular lumen. H&E staining. Magnification 380×.

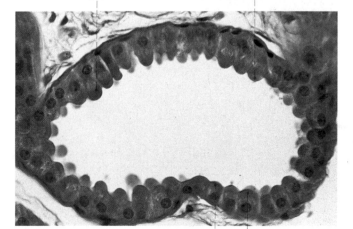

105

Cytoplasmic domes with secretory product

59

Glandular epithelia – Branched and compound glands

Pyloric pit continuing into a simple branched tubular gland

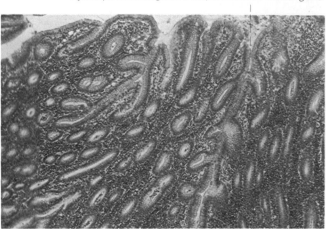

106

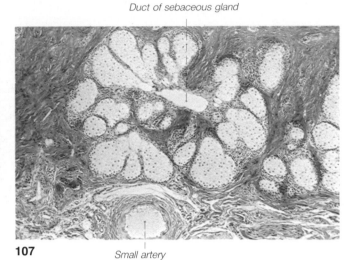

107   *Small artery*

Fig. 106. Simple branched tubular glands from human pyloric antrum. A careful search of the specimen is required to see the tubular shape and branching sites, since only in places do these lie in the plane of the section. H & E staining. Magnification 60×.

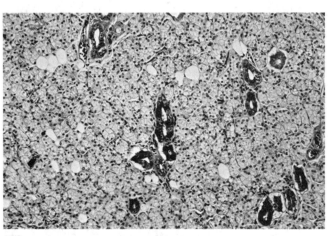

108

Fig. 107. Simple branched alveolar gland (sebaceous gland from human upper eyelid). The lumina of the secretory portions are not visible because most are sectioned tangentially and because they are filled with the holocrine secretory product formed from gradually transforming secretory cells. Mallory-azan staining. Magnification 60×.

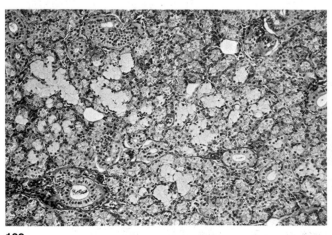

109

Fig. 108. Serous gland (human parotid gland). The nature of the secretory portions indicate that this is an "acinar" gland (cf. Fig. 103) and its elaborately branched duct system shows that it is a "compound" gland. Mallory-azan staining. Magnification 96×.

Fig. 109. Human submandibular gland classified as 1) "mixed" because of the nature of its secretions, 2) "tubulo-acinar" by the arrangement of its secretory units, and 3) "compound" due to its elaborate branching duct. The mucous cells forming the tubular parts of the secretory portions are stained pale blue. Mallory-azan staining. Magnification 96×.

60

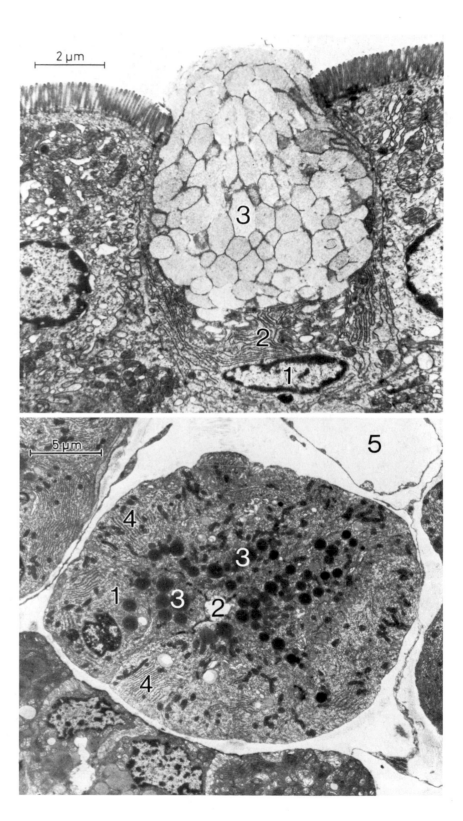

Fig. 110. Goblet cell within the intestinal epithelium of a rat (compare with the light micrographs of Figs. 91 and 100). The bottom of the cell contains the nucleus (**1**) and most of the organelles, particularly a well developed rough ER (**2**). **3** Mucous secretory granules. Magnification 9,000 ×.

Fig. 111. Transverse section of a serous acinus from submucosa of feline nasal septum. The individual cells forming this unit are poorly demarcated and therefore, only one of them (**1**) shows the characteristic wedge-shaped outline. Note the narrow lumen (**2**), the clusters of secretory granules (**3**) and the abluminal concentration of orderly arranged stacks of cisternae of the RER, representing the ultrastructural correlate of the ergastoplasm of light microscopy (**4**). **5** Lumen of fenestrated capillary. Magnification 3,500 ×.

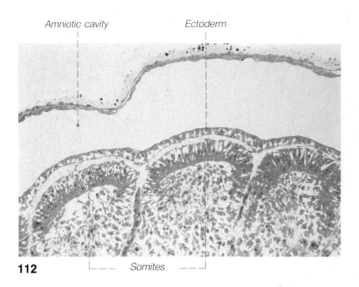

Amniotic cavity   Ectoderm

112   └ ─ ─ Somites ─ ─ ┘

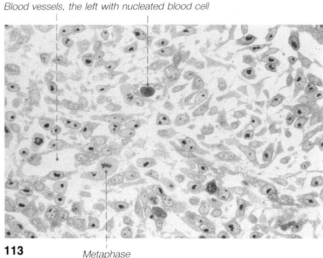

Blood vessels, the left with nucleated blood cell

113   Metaphase

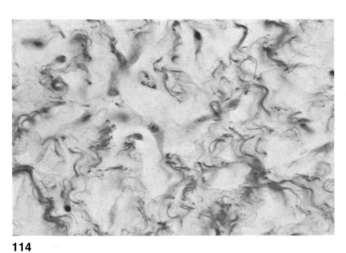

114

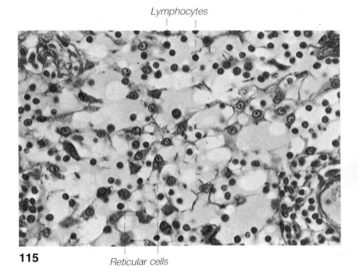

Lymphocytes

115   Reticular cells

Fig. 112. Longitudinal paramedian plastic section (thickness 1 μm) through a chick embryo of four days. Beyond the epithelial surface three somites are clearly outlined that are the source of mobile mesenchymal cells which migrate throughout the developing body to serve as stem cells for all future connective tissue elements. Methylene blue-azure II staining. Magnification 150× (Specimen courtesy of Dr. U. Herrmann, Dept. of Anatomy, Technical University Munich).

Fig. 113. A higher magnification of the mesenchyme illustrates the stellate configuration of its cellular components to better advantage. In addition several mitoses may be seen, together with newly formed blood vessels. The empty spaces are filled *in vivo* with a viscous fluid, the amorphous ground substance. Methylene blue-azure II staining. Magnification 380×.

Fig. 114. Mucous connective tissue with fibers (Wharton's jelly of human umbilical cord). Along with fibroblasts a network of fine collagenous fibers is seen in the amorphous ground substance. Mallory-azan staining. Magnification 380×.

Fig. 115. Reticular connective tissue from a medullary sinus of a cat lymph node. In the center of the micrograph is a network of stellate reticular cells with delicate reticular fibers (stained brilliant blue) closely attached to their surfaces. The many processes of the reticular cells indicate their mesenchymal origin. The round, apparently "naked" nuclei belong to lymphocytes. Mallory-azan staining. Magnification 380×.

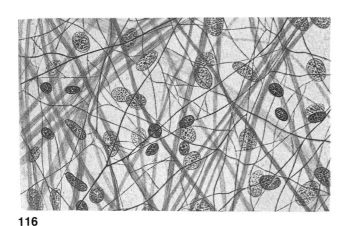

116

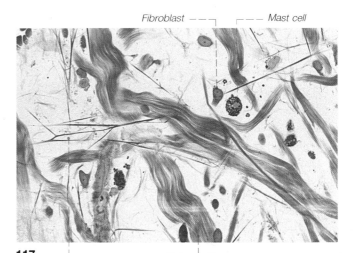

117 *Elastic fiber with branching sites*   *Collagen fiber*

Fibroblast   *Mast cell*

Branching elastic fiber

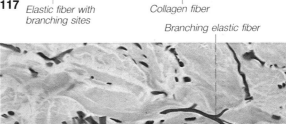

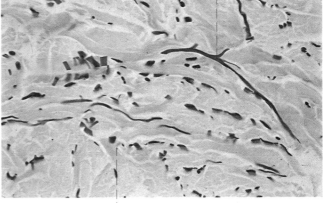

118   *Bundle of collagenous fibers*

Fig. 116. A drawing of a spread- or Häutchen-preparation of loose connective tissue from rat omentum majus. Since the specimen was fixed in a streched state, the collagenous fibers show a straight instead of their usually wavy course (cf. Fig. 117). Collagenous fibers never branch, but they are interwoven, thus forming a loosely arranged feltwork. By contrast, the thin elastic fibers do branch and hence create true networks (cf. Table 7). The 'naked' nuclei belong to the various cellular elements of loose connective tissue. H & E and elastica staining. Magnification approx. 400×.

Fig. 117. Plastic semi-thin (0.5 μm thick) section through rat mesentery clearly illustrates the wavy course of collagenous fibers which also disclose smaller filamentous subunits, i.e. bundles of fibrils. The elastic fibers are the much thinner, more distinctly outlined and branching elements which look like crystalline needles in this preparation. The cells crowded with darkly stained granules represent mast cells, whereas the almost "naked" nuclei belong to fibroblasts. Safranine methylene blue-azure II staining. Magnification 380×.

Fig. 118. Collagen and elastic fibers in human subcutaneous connective tissue. The broad collagen fibers stained pale brown are intersected in all directions by a network of fine elastic fibers (see Table 7). The connective tissue cells are not visible because nuclear counterstaining has not been performed. Resorcin-fuchsin staining. Magnification 240×.

Fig. 119. Reticular fibers shown in the liver by the silver impregnation technique (hence the name "argyrophilic" fibers). These fibers share some of their optical and physicochemical properties with their collagenous counterparts and others with elastic fibers. They are arranged as a delicate filigree-like meshwork at the interface between the interstitial connective tissue (= stroma) and the specific cells (parenchyma) of each organ, forming a mold of their contents, in this case hepatic cells. Bielschowsky's staining. Magnification 240×.

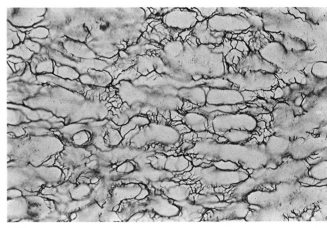

119

Connective tissue – Cell types

Mast cell

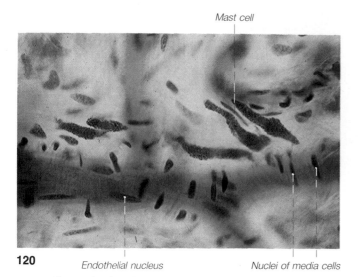

120 Endothelial nucleus   Nuclei of media cells

Serous alveolus

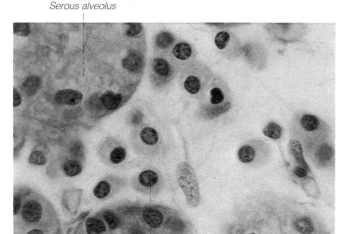

122 Plasma cell

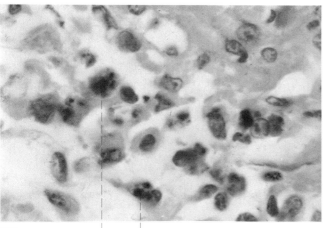

123 Histiocytes

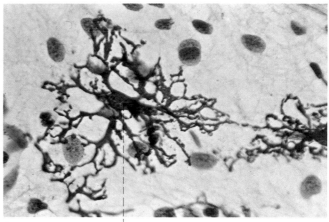

121 Nucleus of pigment cell

Fig. 120. A spread of isolated canine periosteum showing mast cells along a small artery. The mast cells are stained metachromatically due to their high content of heparin, a mucopolysaccharide. Blood vessels injected with a blue gelatin solution. Toluidine blue staining. Magnification 600 ×.

Fig. 121. Richly branched pigment cell (melanocyte or chromatophore) in the subcutaneous tissue of a salamander larva containing large numbers of dark brown or black melanin granules. (In man, skin melanocytes occur only in the epidermal layer). Hematoxylin staining. Magnification 380 ×.

Fig. 122. Plasma cells from the interstitial connective tissue of a human lacrimal gland. A characteristic feature of these cells is their round, eccentrically placed nucleus. The "cartwheel" appearance resulting from regularly arranged chromatin particles within the nucleus is seen much more rarely than is generally believed. The basophilia of the cytoplasm (hence the gray-blue tinge with the azan stain) is due to the abundance of RNA in the form of bound ribosomes on the rough-surfaced endoplasmic reticulum (cf. Fig. 133). Mallory-azan staining. Magnification 960 ×.

Fig. 123. Histiocytes "labeled" by the incorporation of the vital dye trypan blue (loose connective tissue from mouse skin). The high phagocytic activity of motile cells of this type belonging to the reticuloendothelial (mononuclear phagocytic) system, allows for their selective demonstration. Vital staining with trypan blue, counterstained with nuclear fast red. Magnification 960 ×.

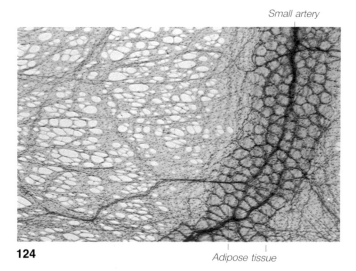

Small artery

124   Adipose tissue

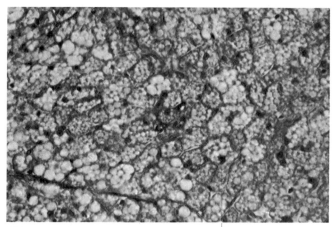

125   Nucleus of a multilocular fat cell

Adipose cell

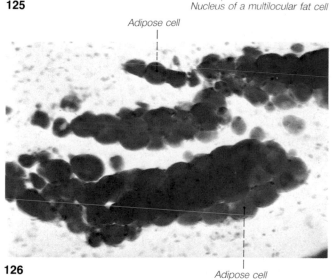

126   Adipose cell

Fig. 124. True areolar connective tissue is found only in the greater and lesser omenta and some of the mesenteries. The many empty elliptical spaces are not fat cells, but represent true cavities surrounded by a connective tissue framework that is covered by a mesothelial layer. On the right side, a branching artery embedded in adipose tissue can be seen. Hematoxylin and benzo light Bordeaux staining. Magnification 38×.

Fig. 125. Multilocular adipose tissue from a cat fetus. As the name indicates, each cell contains several fat droplets that gradually coalesce to result finally in one large droplet almost completely filling the cell body (see also Fig. 134). In this case many of the nuclei are pushed to the periphery although they still preserve their spherical shape. Mallory-azan staining. Magnification 240×.

Fig. 126. Small lobules of adipose tissue from rat mesentery. The individual fat cells are often ill defined because each is closely attached and partly overlaps its neighbor. In this preparation the lipid droplet that almost completely fills the cell body has been preserved and selectively stained. Hemalum and Sudan red staining. Magnification 150×.

Fig. 127. Adipose tissue from a human lacrimal gland. Since fat is dissolved out by the alcohol, benzene, etc., used for tissue dehydration prior to paraffin or celloidin embedding, the cells appear as empty profiles. The boundaries of these spaces are not the cell membrane, but consist of the plasmalemma and a thin rim of cytoplasm displaced to the cell periphery by the large fat droplets. The nuclei are flattened and usually found pressed against the cell wall. Mallory-azan staining. Magnification 150×.

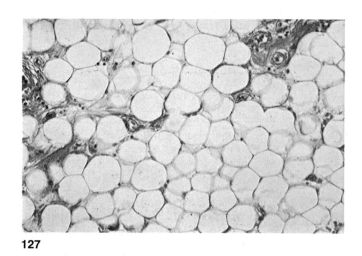

127

Collagenous fibers – Electron microscopy

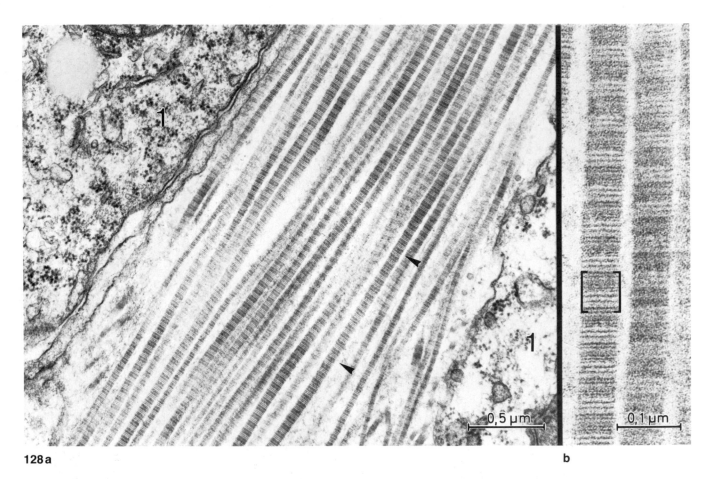

128a   **b**

Fig. 128. a) A small bundle of longitudinally sectioned collagen fibrils lying between fibroblasts (**1**) in Syrian hamster subcutaneous tissue. Note characteristic cross-striation with major axial repeating units (one light and one electron dense band) at every 67 nm. Both parts of such a period are subdivided by additional dark lines of which those bisecting the light bands (►) are particularly prominent. Magnification 39,000 ×.

b) A higher resolution depicts finer details of the banded pattern of a single collagen fibril disclosing at least 6–8 delicate electron dense lines within each period ([ ]). Magnification 160,000 ×.

Fig. 129. Richly vascularized loose connective tissue from cat submandibular gland. Numerous elongated slender whip-like cytoplasmic processes (**1**) only occasionally show their origin from the cell bodies (**2₁, 2₂**) of fibroblasts. **3₁** and **3₂** = Lumina of postcapillary venules; **4** = Bundle of cross-sectioned collagen fibrils. Magnification 8,000 ×.

Fig. 130. a) b) Parts of the perikarya of a fibrocyte (**a**) and a fibroblast (**b**), each containing the nucleus and the majority of the organelles. The fibroblast can be identified as such by its well-developed and evidently highly active rough endoplasmic reticulum (**1**) together with the numerous Golgi complexes (**2**) indicative of synthetic processes. **3** = Non-myelinated nerve. Magnification 14,500 × and 10,500 ×.

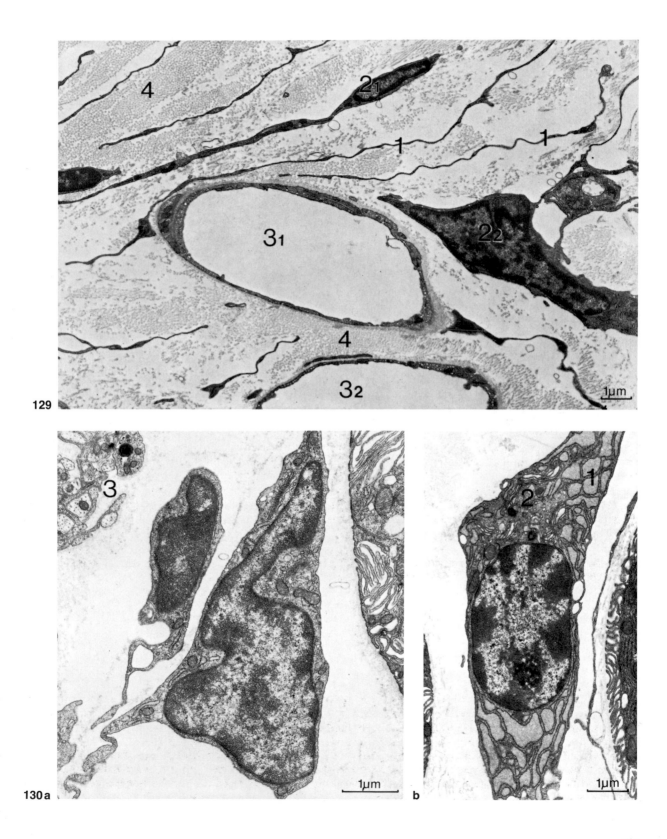

Connective tissue, cell types – Electron microscopy

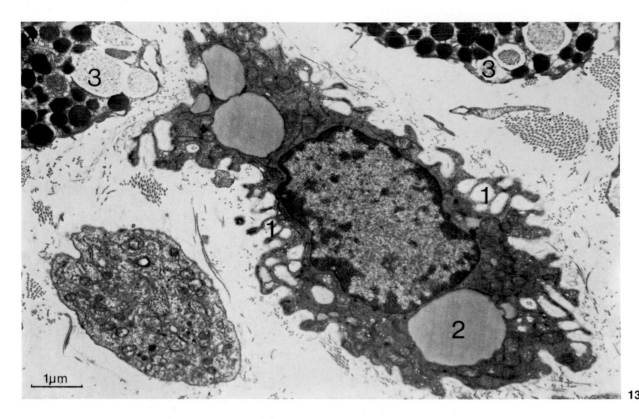

Fig. 131.   Histiocyte from rat subcutaneous connective tissue. The fine structure of these ameboid and highly phagocytic cells is characterized by an intensely vacuolated outer cytoplasmic fringe (**1**) that corresponds to the many pseudopod-like processes. Besides the usual organelles, the cell body may contain a large variety of inclusion bodies originating from the enzymatic breakdown of phagocytized materials into secondary lysosomes and residual bodies. However, in this case the histiocyte only contains lipid droplets (**2**) of different sizes. **3** Parts of a mast cell. Magnification 13,000×.

Fig. 132. a)   Mast cell from loose connective tissue of Syrian hamster cheek pouch. Characteristic of this mobile type of cells are the large, globular, and membrane-bound granules of varying electron opacity (**1, 2, 3**). These correspond to different stages of maturity of these corpuscles which store, amongst other substances histamine and heparin. Note also the numerous slender processes projecting from the cell surface. Magnification 20,000×.

b)   Part of a human mast cell from submucosa of renal pelvis to illustrate characteristic granules displaying membranous scrolls (**1**) and denser cores (**2**) together with other lamellar contents (**3**). Magnification 43,000×.

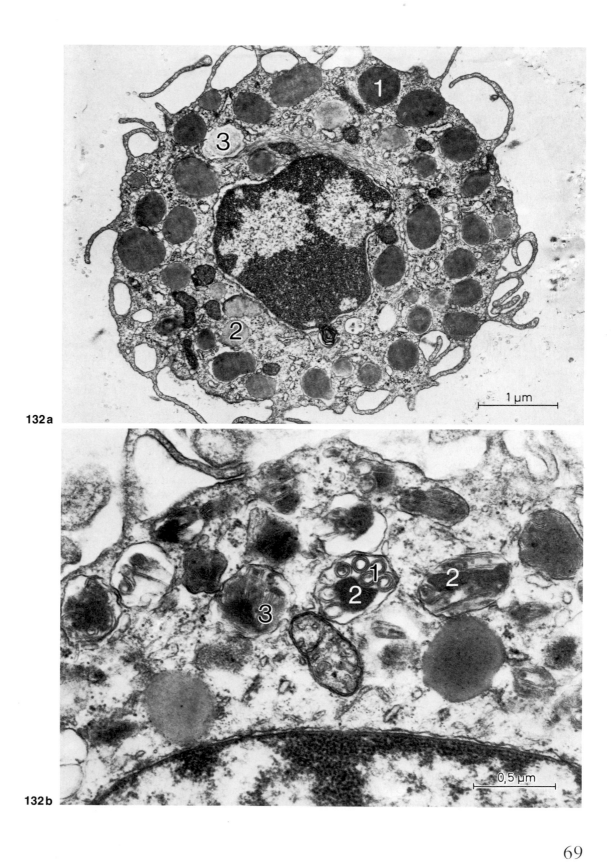

132a

1 µm

132b

0,5 µm

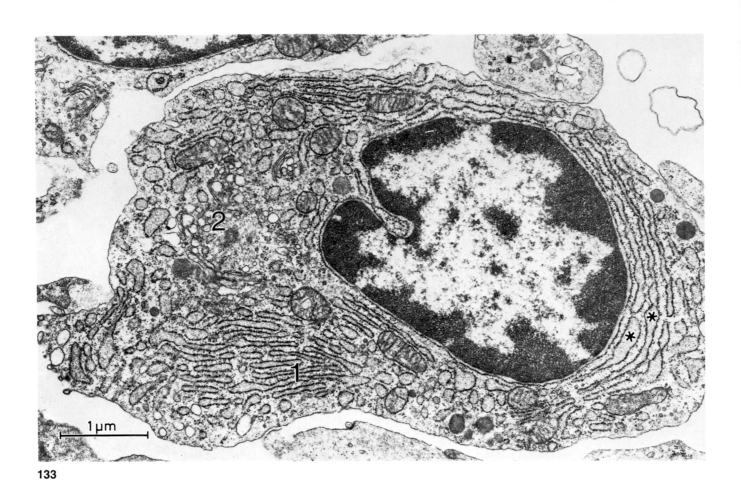

133

Fig. 133. Plasma cell from rat intestinal submucosa. These cells belong to the facultative cellular components of loose connective tissue and they are characterized by an abundance of RER (**1**) that serves for the synthesis of immune globulins. The cisternae of RER are moderately expanded at (∗) and they are all filled with a finely flocculent, most probably proteinaceous material. **2** Golgi apparatus. Magnification 22,000 ×.

Fig. 134. Multilocular fat cell from rat subcutaneous tissue. The cell is filled with five large lipid inclusions (**1**), some of which (★) are incompletely separated by an extremely fine discontinuous cytoplasmic partition (►). The remaining cytoplasm of this young adipose cell (adipocyte) appears rather electron dense and contains, besides the nucleus (**2**), several smaller vacuoles (→). Magnification 4,000 ×.

Fig. 135. Portions of two chondrocytes from mouse elastic cartilage. The two cells are closely attached to each other and both reveal dilated cisternae of their rough ER (∗) indicative for the synthesis of 'proteins for export'. In this case production of the precursors for collagen fibrils and the amorphous ground substance. Magnification 14,000 ×.

70

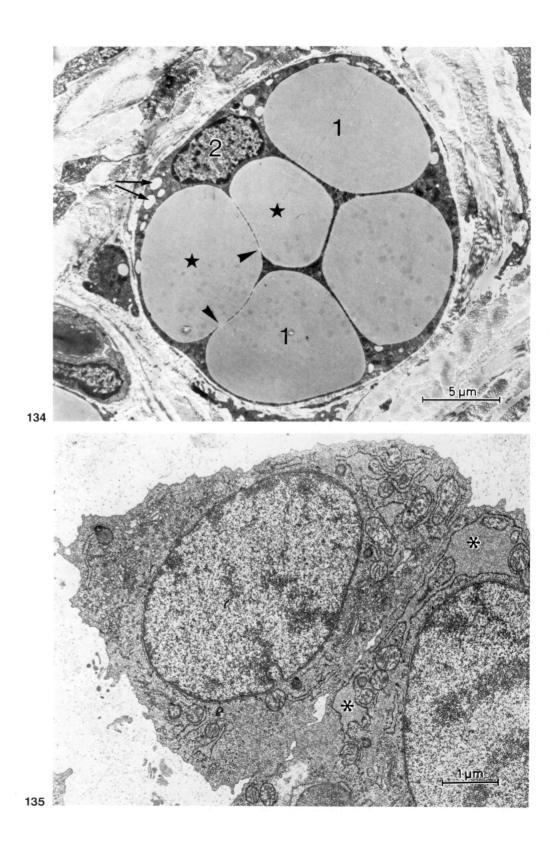

134

135

Loose connective tissue

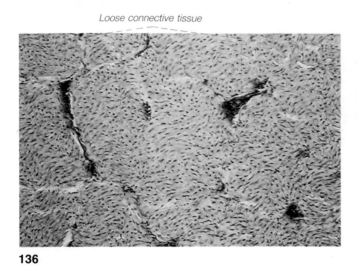

136

Strand of loose connective tissue

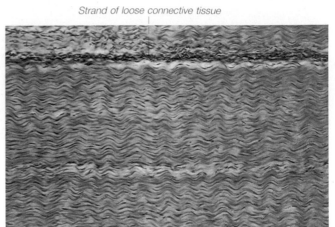

137

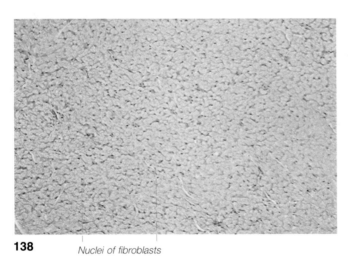

138   *Nuclei of fibroblasts*

139

Fig. 136. Cross-sectioned canine tendon clearly showing its subdivision into smaller fiber bundles by strands of loose connective tissue. Note the large number of fibroblast nuclei, found in almost every interstice between the tendon fibers. A similar though less obvious appearance is seen in longitudinal section (see Fig. 137). H & E staining. Magnification 95 ×.

Fig. 137. Longitudinal section of the same tendon shown in Figure 136. Note fibroblasts arranged in parallel rows with only their nuclei visible. The undulating appearance is one characteristic of tendon fibers but this is not the sole criterion for identification since it is shared by longitudinally sectioned nerve trunks. A strand of loose connective tissue crosses the upper part of the micrograph. H & E staining. Magnification 95 ×.

Fig. 138. Cross-section of an elastic ligament (bovine nuchal ligament). In this photomicrograph the elastic fibers are stained yellowish-green (with azan or eosin methylene blue they would stain brilliant red) and the sparse delicate collagen fibers are blue to bluish-green. The majority of the nuclei present throughout the section belong to fibroblasts, which are found in association with both elastic and collagenous elements (cf. Fig. 136). Iron hematoxylin and picroindigocarmine staining. Magnification 95 ×.

Fig. 139. Longitudinal section of the same specimen shown in Figure 138. Note the small number of nuclei and the broad partly parallel elastic fibers. The fibers branch often and fuse at acute angles like in a stretched fishing net (cf. Fig. 137). Iron hematoxylin and picroindigocarmine staining. Magnification 95 ×.

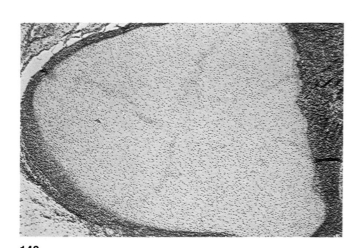

140

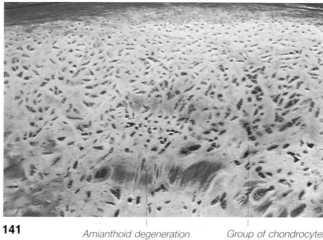

141   *Amianthoid degeneration*   *Group of chondrocytes*

Fig. 140.   Fetal hyaline cartilage from human calcaneus. Note that the numerous cartilage cells are disposed diffusely throughout the tissue rather than in groups and that the matrix appears homogeneous and stains uniformly. (cf. Fig. 141). Mallory-azan staining. Magnification 38 ×.

Fig. 141.   Mature hyaline cartilage from human rib at a low magnification. The cells (= chondrocytes) are arranged in groups and the matrix stains variably, showing the heterogeneous distribution of the different components of the intercellular material. In the lower part of the micrograph a typical degenerative alteration of hyaline cartilage can be seen. Known as amianthoid degeneration, this arises by a change in the chemical composition of the ground substance allowing its tightly packed collagen fiber content to become visible. H & E staining. Magnification 38 ×.

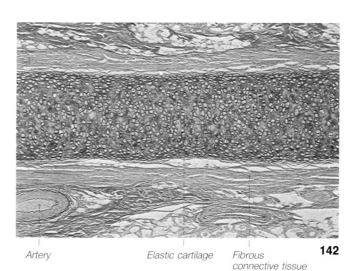

Artery   *Elastic cartilage*   *Fibrous* **142**
              connective tissue

Fig. 142.   Elastic cartilage from the external ear of a pig. The cartilage cells, scattered regularly throughout the matrix, are often found in groups of two, which are infrequently seen in hyaline cartilage. The intercellular material is colored dark reddish-violet due to selective staining of its elastic network by resorcin-fuchsin. At this low magnification individual elastic fibers are not visualized (cf. Fig. 146).Resorcin-fuchsin, nuclear fast red staining. Magnification 38 ×.

Fig. 143.   Fibrous cartilage (= fibrocartilage) from human intervertebral disk. In this type of cartilage the collagen fibers are not masked and thus always visible, often arranged in a characteristic herringbone pattern. The matrix contains only a few, usually singly distributed cells, hardly visible at this low magnification. H & E staining. Magnification 38 ×.

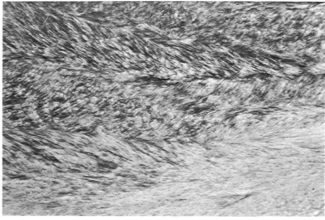

143

Connective tissue – Cartilage

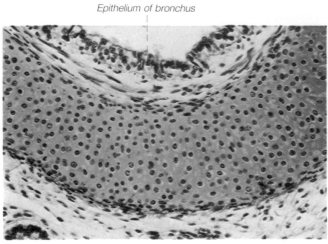

144

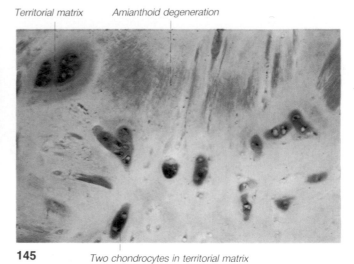

145   *Two chondrocytes in territorial matrix*

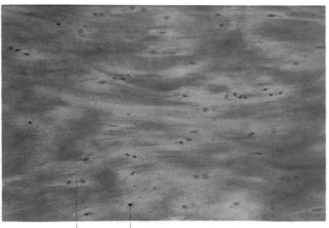

146   *Bicellular groups of chondrocytes*

Fig. 144. Hyaline cartilage from the bronchus of a human fetal lung. The singly distributed chondrocytes have nearly circular cellular and nuclear outlines and are embedded in a homogeneous matrix. Mallory-azan staining. Magnification 240×.

Fig. 145. Mature hyaline cartilage from human rib (higher magnification of part of Fig. 141) showing amianthoid degeneration and groups of rather small chondrocytes. The translucent spaces are lacunae in which the cells are located. During histological processing the cells shrink considerably into small masses in which often only the nuclei are visible, showing as densely stained structures. The basophilic areas surrounding each cell group are known as "capsules" and consist of parts of the territorial matrix particularly rich in glycosaminoglycans. H&E staining. Magnification 150×.

Fig. 146. Elastic cartilage from the external ear of a pig (same specimen as in Fig. 142), the chondrocytes of which are considerably less shrunken than those in Figure 145. Their nuclei (stained pale pink) have thus maintained their spherical shape and are haloed by the weaker staining of the cell body. Due to shrinkage the cells have separated from the lacunar walls. Note the bicellular groups of chondrocytes and the dense network of elastic fibers. Resorcin-fuchsin, nuclear fast red staining. Magnification 150×.

Fig. 147. Fibrocartilage from human intervertebral disk. The uni- or bicellular groups of chondrocytes are irregularly distributed between the collagen fiber bundles of the matrix and only their nuclei are clearly recognizable. H&E staining. Magnification 150×.

147   *Cartilage cells in hyaline matrix*

Hair germ   Epidermis   Blood vessels

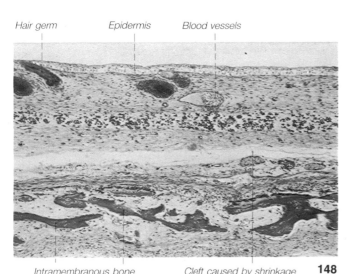

Intramembranous bone   Cleft caused by shrinkage   **148**

Osteoblasts

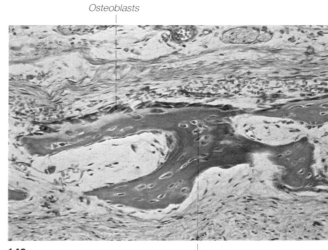

149

Osteocytes
Osteoblasts

Fig. 148. Human fetal cranium as an example of intramembranous bone development in which mesenchymal cells transform into osteoblasts, the latter producing the non-calcified osseous ground substance or osteoid. Some of the osteoblasts become surrounded by osteoid and, with the deposition of calcium salts into the osteoid, become osteocytes as the osteoid progressively hardens around them. H & E staining. Magnification 38×.

Fig. 149. A close-up of the lower right corner of Figure 148 clearly illustrates osteoblasts closely attached to the surface of, and osteocytes located within, the osseous trabeculae. H & E staining. Magnification 150×.

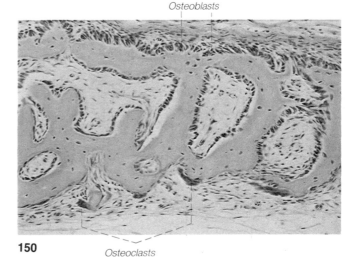

150   Osteoclasts

Osteoblasts

Fig. 150. Trabeculae from canine fetal mandible. The osseous surfaces oriented towards the skin are covered with osteoblasts, the source of osteoid, while those facing the oral cavity show osteoclasts (a type of multinucleate giant cell) that are responsible for the enzymatic resorption of bone. H & E staining. Magnification 95×.

Fig. 151. Fetal skull of a pig, the osseous trabeculae (stained blue) of which are covered by numerous osteoblasts responsible for the growth of the bone by the apposition of more and more ground substance. At the same time enzymatic resorption is occurring on the inner surface because of the osteoclasts. Small recesses (= Howship's lacunae) are formed in which the osteoclasts are often found. The apposition of bone on the outer surface and its resorption on the inner surface serves to enlarge the cranium and thus to accommodate the rapidly developing brain. Mallory-azan staining. Magnification 240×.

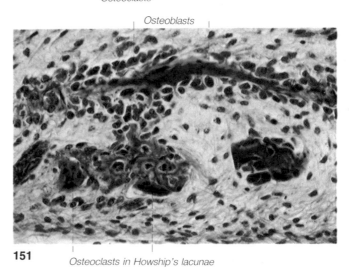

151   Osteoclasts in Howship's lacunae

Connective tissue – Development and growth of bone

Fig. 152. Early stage of intracartilaginous osteogenesis in a phalanx of a three-month-old human fetus. In contrast to intramembranous bone development, this form of ossification starts with a cartilaginous model of the later bone that is resorbed and then gradually replaced by osseous tissue. The process begins near the middle of the future shaft with calcification of the cartilaginous ground substance to form the diaphyseal or primary ossification center. This is accompanied by proliferation and hypertrophy of local chondrocytes and by the deposition of a bony collar around the cartilage of the ossification center. The latter is known as perichondral ossification because the bone is derived from osteoblasts that develop from mesenchymal cells in the perichondrium. Note that, despite the different terminology, the basic mechanisms by which osseous tissue is formed is the same in both intramembranous and intracartilaginous ossification (camera lucida drawing). H & E staining. Magnification 80 ×.

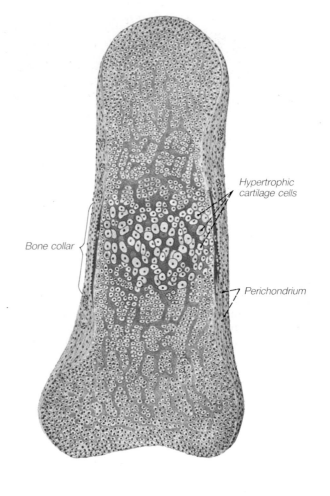

Hypertrophic cartilage cells

Bone collar

Perichondrium

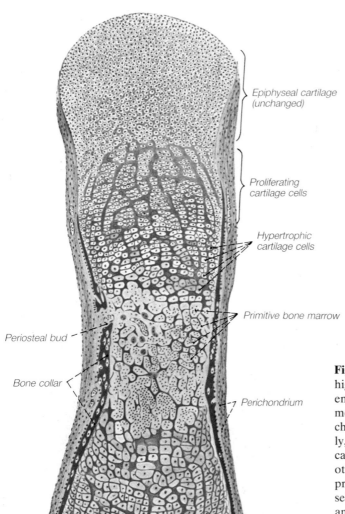

Epiphyseal cartilage (unchanged)

Proliferating cartilage cells

Hypertrophic cartilage cells

Primitive bone marrow

Periosteal bud

Bone collar

Perichondrium

Fig. 153. In a second phase periosteal buds, representing a highly vascular mesenchyme, grow through the bony collar and enter the periphery of the primary ossification center. This mesenchyme contains chondroclasts and osteogenic cells. The chondroclasts resorb the calcified cartilage matrix enzymatically, transforming the hypertrophied lacunae into a system of cavities, the primary marrow spaces. The spaces are filled with other elements of the actively proliferating mesenchyme, the primary bone marrow, from which osteoblasts attach themselves to the surfaces of the residual calcified cartilage matrix and begin to cover these trabeculae with osteoid (camera lucida drawing). H & E staining. Magnification 100 ×.

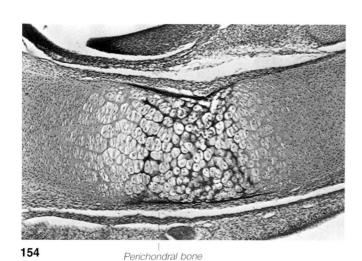

154   *Perichondral bone*

Calcified cartilagineous ground substance

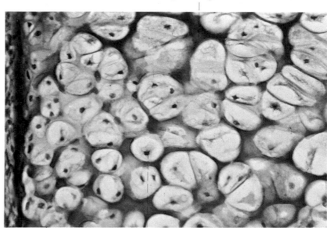

Perichondral bone   *Nucleus of a shrunken chondrocyte*   **155**
Epiphyseal cartilage   *Primitive bone marrow*

Fig. 154. Longitudinal section through a metacarpal bone from a human fetus. Centrally the chondrocytes are hypertrophied and the adjacent cartilage matrix has been calcified, rendering it more basophilic. This process establishes the primary ossification center. H & E staining. Magnification 60 ×.

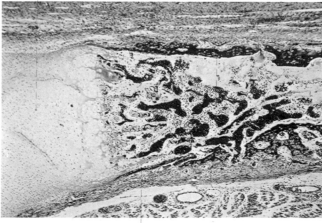

Fig. 155. A close-up of the primary ossification center from the preceding micrograph clearly shows the enlargement of the lacunae that is caused by considerable swelling of the chondrocytes. Details of this cellular degeneration, however, are not seen because of the shrinkage artifact that often occurs during routine histologic preparation. H & E staining. Magnification 240 ×.

156   *Perichondral bone*

Blood vessels stuffed with erythrocytes

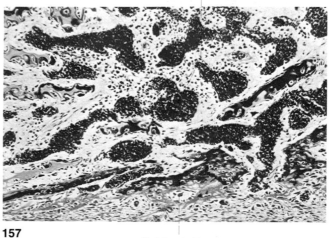

Fig. 156. Longitudinal section through a metatarsal bone from an 18-cm human fetus that matches the camera lucida drawing of Figure 158. Mallory-azan staining. Magnification 38 ×.

Fig. 157. A close-up of the lower part of the preceding micrograph reveals numerous openings in the perichondral bone collar through which mesenchyme, including blood vessels, enters the primary marrow cavity. Mallory-azan staining. Magnification 96 ×.

157   *Perichondral bone*

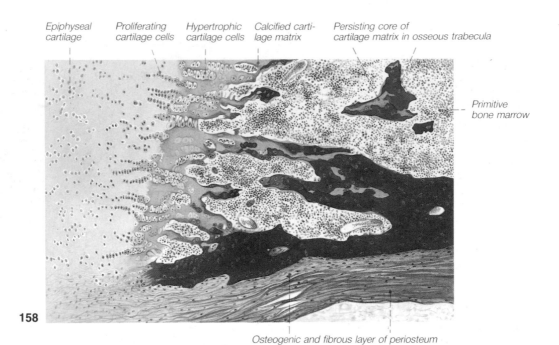

Epiphyseal cartilage — Proliferating cartilage cells — Hypertrophic cartilage cells — Calcified cartilage matrix — Persisting core of cartilage matrix in osseous trabecula

Primitive bone marrow

158

Osteogenic and fibrous layer of periosteum

Fig. 158. Detail from a third and later stage of intracartilaginous bone development. The marrow cavity has enlarged considerably towards the epiphyseal ends where it reaches the hyaline cartilage, which shows calcification (and thus increased basophilia) of its matrix along with cellular hypertrophy. Note that the same degenerative processes precede the resorption of the cartilage here as already described for the formation of the primary ossification center (see Fig. 152). Remnants of the original calcified cartilage ground substance allow the early attachment of osteoblasts, thus serving as guidelines for ossification and as a supporting framework that persists for some time (camera lucida drawing). H&E staining. Magnification 80×.

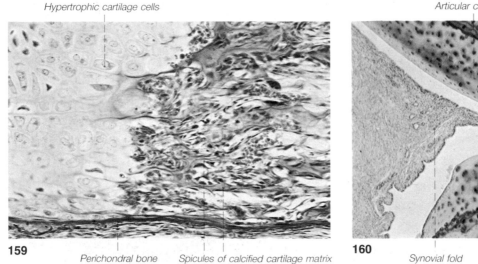

Hypertrophic cartilage cells

159

Perichondral bone   Spicules of calcified cartilage matrix

Fig. 159. Border zone between epiphyseal cartilage and marrow cavity from the proximal third of a human fetal humerus. Remnants of the calcified cartilage matrix (colored violet) project like spicules from the zone of hypertrophied cartilage into the highly cellular and intensely vascularized marrow cavity. H&E staining. Magnification 150×.

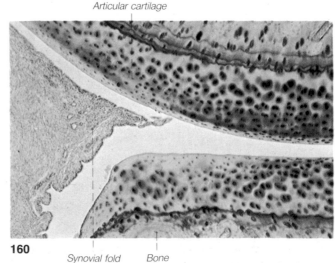

Articular cartilage

160

Synovial fold   Bone

Fig. 160. Part of a section from a human fetal knee joint. Even at this early stage the cells of the articular cartilage, a derivative of the epiphyseal cartilage, are clearly divided into small groups. On the left a synovial villus protrudes into the joint cavity. H&E staining. Magnification 38×.

78

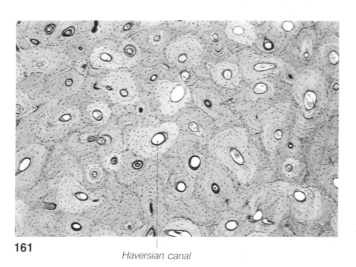

161   *Haversian canal*

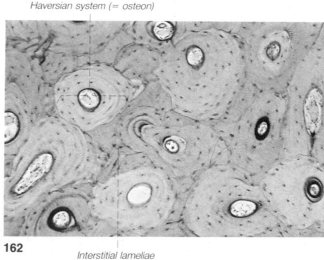

Haversian system (= osteon)

162   *Interstitial lameliae*

Fig. 161 and 162. Transverse section through the compact bone of a human fibula showing numerous Haversian systems, each of which consists of several osseous lamellae concentrically arranged around a circular opening, the Haversian canal. A higher magnification (Fig. 162) reveals the osteocytes as darker colored dots wedged in between the osseous lamellae and aligned in concentric circular lines. Remnants of former Haversian systems constitute the interstitial lamellae filling the spaces between the osteons. Fuchsin staining. Magnification 38× and 96×.

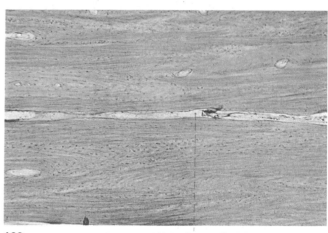

163   *Haversian canal*

Fig. 163. Longitudinal section through the compact bone of a canine humerus. In the center is a Haversian canal. In contrast to ground bone preparations as shown in Figure 164 real sections of decalcified bone always show the loose connective tissue in the Haversian canals and the endosteum as well as other remnants of connective tissue like the periosteum. Carbolthionine staining. Magnification 38×.

Lacuna   *Canaliculi*

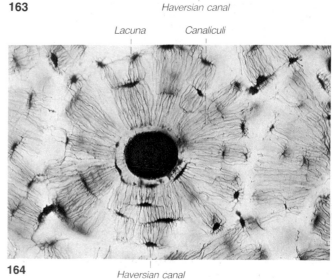

Fig. 164. Ground bone preparation from the shaft of a canine femur. When these paper-thin slices – prepared by grinding down a piece of bone using abrasives – are stained, the elliptical cavities (= lacunae) and delicate canaliculi, which housed the osteocyte cell bodies and their processes, are clearly outlined. The lacunae are always arrayed parallel to, and the canaliculi perpendicular to, the lamellae. Fuchsin staining. Magnification 240×.

164   *Haversian canal*

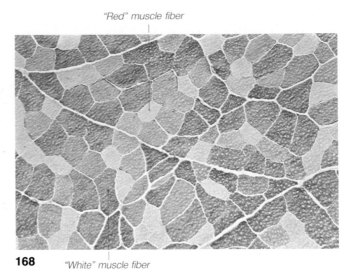

"Red" muscle fiber

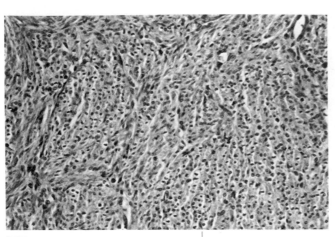

165

Apparently "naked" nuclei of smooth muscle cells

168

"White" muscle fiber

Myofibrillae-free sarcoplasmic area

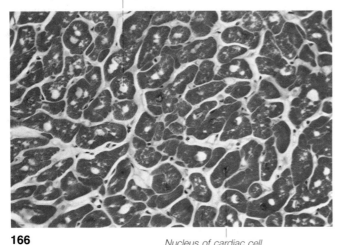

Fig. 168. Demonstration of three different types of skeletal muscle fibers by their varying glycogen content (rat anterior tibialis muscle). The "red" fibers with an extremely low content of glycogen are nearly unstained, the intermediate type fibers are moderately colored and the glycogen-rich "white" fibers stain a brilliant magenta. PAS staining. Magnification 96 ×.

166

Nucleus of cardiac cell

Nucleus of skeletal muscle fiber

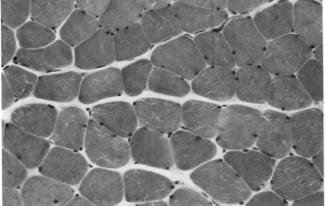

Fig. 165–167. The three types of muscular tissue all illustrated in transverse sections with the same stain (H & E) and magnification (240 ×).

Despite the fact that the nuclei are not very prominent at this magnification, the different sizes of the cross-sectional areas of muscle *cells* (human uterine smooth muscle, Fig. 165, and canine myocardium, Fig. 166), and of muscle *fibers* (human sternohyoid muscle, Fig. 167) are a helpful criterion for distinguishing the three muscle tissues one from another. Compare with the matching longitudinal sections in Figures 170–172. The "empty" spaces in many of the cardiac cells correspond to the myofibril-free axial sarcoplasmic areas located at the nuclear poles.

167

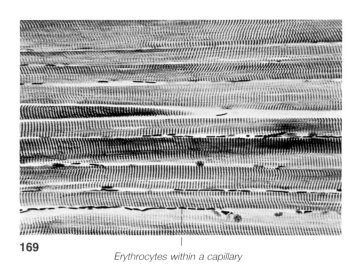

169

Erythrocytes within a capillary

Fig. 169. Special stains like iron hematoxylin are often used to demonstrate cross-striations particularly clearly, thus allowing certain indentification of the A- and I-bands even at rather low magnifications (canine hyoid muscle). The bluish-black structures aligned parallel to the edges of the fibers are not the nuclei of the muscle fibers, but erythrocytes compressed within narrow capillaries. Iron hematoxylin staining.   Magnification 240×.

Small bundles of smooth muscle cells

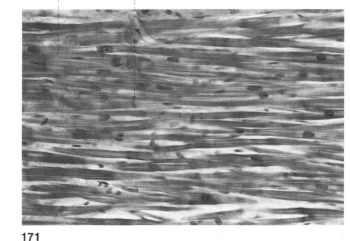

170   *Small vein*

Cross-striation   *Intercalated disk*

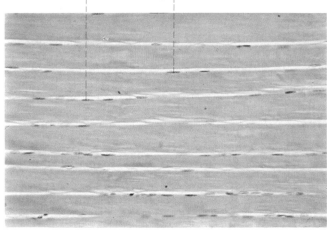

171

Nuclei of skeletal muscle fibers

Figs. 170–172.   The three types of muscular tissue all illustrated in longitudinal sections with the same stain (H & E) and magnification (× 240).
Note the axial position of the nuclei in both smooth muscle (human myometrium, Fig. 170) and cardiac cells (canine myocardium, Fig. 171). In muscle fibers (canine hyoid muscle, Fig. 172), the nuclei are located directly below the sarcolemma and occur in very large numbers within each fiber. Cross-striations are barely visible in both the skeletal and cardiac muscle tissues, as are the intercalated disks in the myocardium.

172

Muscular tissue

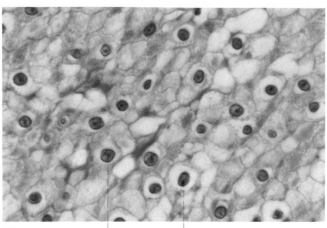

173   *Nuclei of smooth muscle cells*

The three different structural elements found in muscle tissues demonstrated in transverse sections with the same stain (Mallory-azan) and with identical high resolution (× 100 oil immersion objective) and magnification (× 960) for better identification of cytological details.

Fig. 173.   Smooth muscle cells from the muscularis externa of a human vermiform appendix. Note the axial position of the nuclei and the surrounding pale rim of cytoplasm.

A single cardiac cell

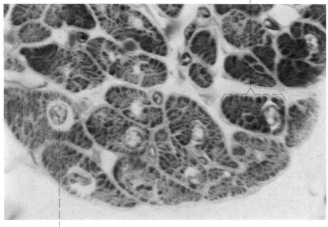

174   *Nucleus surrounded by myofibrillae-free sarcoplasm*

Fig. 174.   Cardiac muscle cells have a notably larger and more irregular cross-sectional area than smooth muscle cells. Their myofibrils are often arranged in small groups, known as Cohnheim fields, separated by narrow strands of sarcoplasm.

Erythrocyte within a capillary

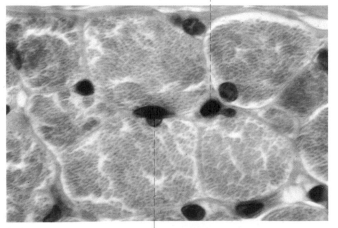

175   *Nucleus of skeletal muscle fiber*

Fig. 175.   Clearly visible myofibrils in skeletal muscle fibers from human orbicularis oculi muscle.

82

The three different structural elements found in muscle tissues demonstrated in longitudinal sections with the same stain (Mallory-azan) and with identical high resolution (× 100 oil immersion objective) and magnification (× 960) for better identification of cytological details.

Nucleus of smooth muscle cell

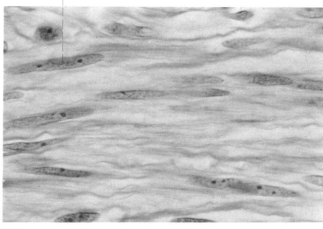

176

Fig. 176. Smooth muscle cells from the muscularis externa of a human vermiform appendix. Although the elongated nuclei with their prominent nucleoli are clearly visible, the cell boundaries are poorly defined, a normal feature of longitudinally sectioned smooth muscle due to the delicacy of its cells.

Intercalated disks

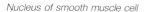

Fig. 177. Cardiac muscle cells from a dog. The sarcoplasmic areas at the nuclear poles are free of myofibrils, but contain lipofuscin granules. Note the darker-red intercalated disks that serve for the cohesion of successive cells and the cross- and longitudinal striation of the cells due to the arrangement of their myofibrils.

Nucleus with nucleolus   *Lipofuscin granules*   **177**

A-band   *Z-line*

Fig. 178. Skeletal muscle fibers with prominent cross-striations from human pectoralis major muscle. The near identical width of the lighter I- (= isotropic) and darker A- (=anisotropic) bands indicates that the muscle has been fixed in a largely relaxed state. Note the prominent Z-lines in the middle of each of the I-bands. (The M- and H-bands contained within the A-bands are not seen here). Directly subjacent to the sarcolemma, two nuclei with nucleoli are faintly visible.

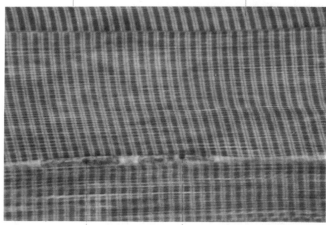

178   *Nucleoli*

Muscular tissue

Bundles of smooth muscle cells

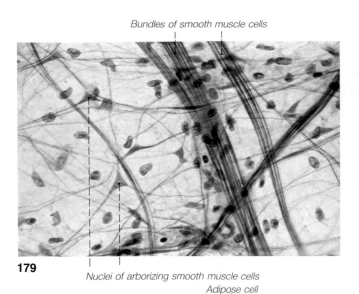

179

Nuclei of arborizing smooth muscle cells

Adipose cell

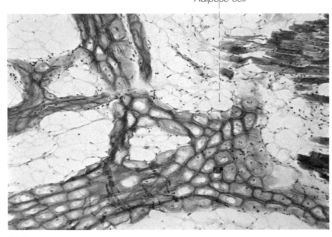

180a

Ordinary cardiac muscle

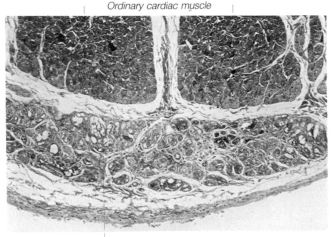

180b   Small bundle of Purkinje fibers

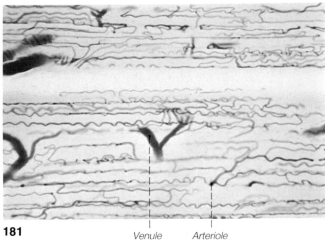

181   Venule   Arteriole

Fig. 179. Arborizing smooth muscle cells with prominent triangular nuclei in a thin spread of a frog urinary bladder. The rest of the muscle is arranged in bundles of long slender cells in which the nuclei are barely visible. H & E staining. Magnification 240 ×.

Figs. 180. a) b) Purkinje fibers of the heart (dog and man) shown in longitudinal and transverse section with the same stain (Mallory-azan) and magnification (× 96). These ultimate branches of the impulse conducting system are composed of highly specialized cardiac cells that are distinguished from ordinary cardiac muscle cells by their larger size, their smaller nuclei, their higher glycogen content and their fewer myofibrils, the latter arranged at the cell periphery. Purkinje fibers form only a small proportion of the total cardiac cell population and are thus seen infrequently in histological sections.

Fig. 181. Vascular injection specimen of a canine skeletal muscle to show the arrangement of its microvasculature. The wavy, tortuous course of the capillaries is not due to muscular contractions, nor is it a means to accommodate variations in fiber length, but a characteristic feature of capillaries supplying "red" fibers. Injection with a gelatin solution colored with carmine, no counterstain. Magnification 96 ×.

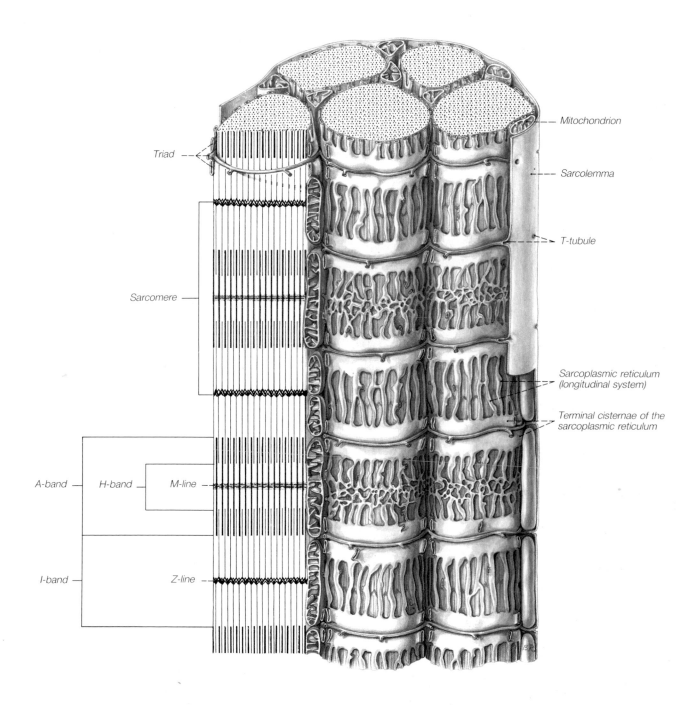

Fig. 182. Schematic three-dimensional representation of the interrelationships of the sarcoplasmic reticulum (= longitudinal system), the T-tubules (= transverse system) and the myofibrils in a mammalian skeletal muscle fiber. Each triad consists of a centrally positioned T-tubule flanked by two terminal cisternae of the sarcoplasmic reticulum that appear as translucent vacuoles in ultra-thin sections. In mammalian muscles the triads are situated at the *A – I* junction, so that there are two triads in each sarcomere along every myofibril (drawing by Mrs. B. Ruppel, Munich, FRG).

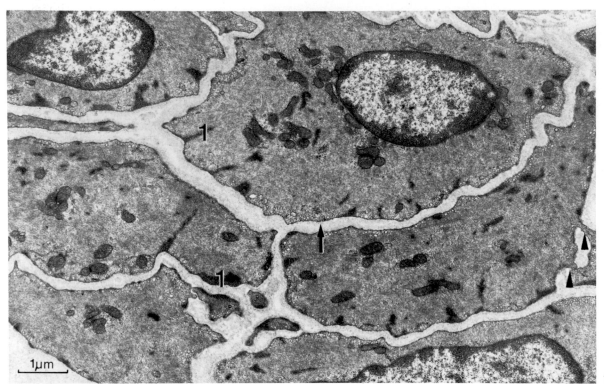

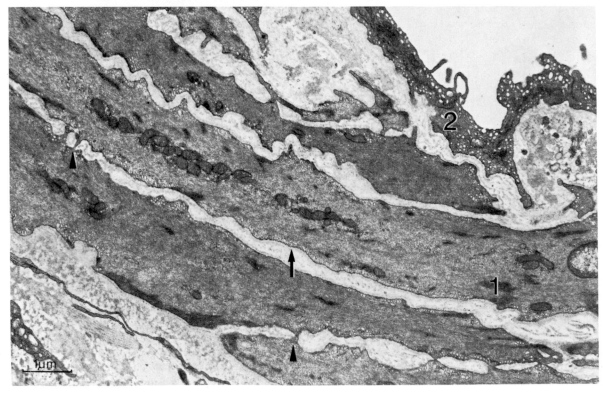

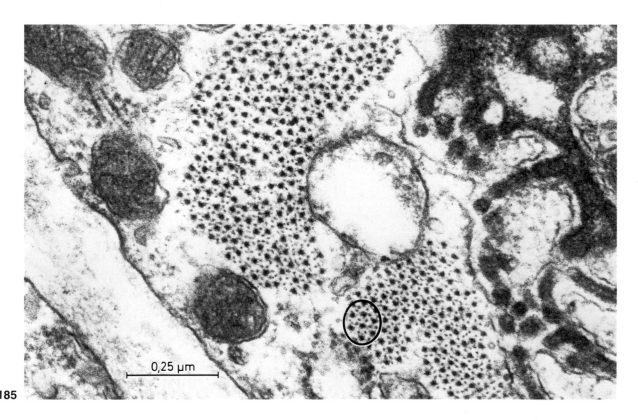

185

Fig. 185. In favorable sections, smooth muscle cells (from rat portal vein) also display thin and thick filaments arranged in a regular pattern, six thin filaments surrounding each of the thick filaments. This special arrangement results in a precise hexagonal array of the myosin filaments that are positioned at the angles of the hexagons (circled). Magnification 96,000 ×.

Figs. 183, 184. Electron micrographs of smooth muscle cells from the media of a small artery in a cat. The size and appearance of the cells vary widely depending on the point of section through the cell and on the number and shape of their cytoplasmic projections. The cell body is largely filled with filamentous material of uniform density (myofilaments) so that the mitochondria and other organelles tend to be located close to the nucleus. The oval or fusiform densities, so-called dense bodies (**1**), found mainly along the inner aspect of the cell membrane, serve as attachment sites for the contractile elements. Muscle cells make numerous close intercelluar contacts by means of small pleomorphic projections (▶) that display gap junctions (= nexus) at the cellular interface. Gap junctions are known to be sites of low electric resistance allowing the intramural spread of excitation from one cell to another. The membrane vesicles or caveolae arranged either in rows or in small groups (→) serve as stores for calcium ions. Because of this function and their close relationship with the poorly developed ER, these vesicles may correspond to the T-tubules of skeletal and cardiac muscle. **2** Endothelium. Magnification 13,000 ×.

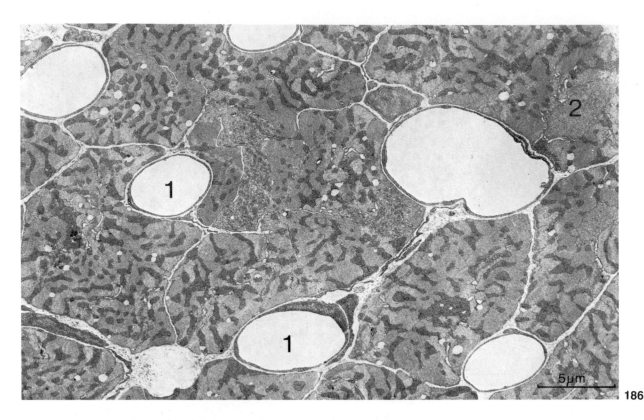

Fig. 186. Transverse section of a feline papillary muscle to show the characteristic variations in size and shape of the individual cross-sectioned cardiac cells which are often rather poorly delineated. Note the close relationship between capillaries (**1**) and muscle cells. **2** Nucleus of a cardiac cell. Magnification 4,000 ×.

Fig. 187. Oblique section through the myocardium of a pig clearly showing the A- and I-bands and Z-lines of its cross-banding. The individual myocardial cells are difficult to distinguish from each other due to their close apposition, but the capillaries (**1**) are helpful for the detection of the narrow interstitial spaces. **2** Nuclei of a cardiac cells. Magnification 4,000 ×.

Fig. 188. Parts of two cardiomyocytes from guinea pig heart joining in an intercalated disk. The apposing cell membranes pursue a wavy course but remain parallel to each other. The subsarcolemmal cytoplasm displays diffuse as well as circumscribed densities (→) similar to desmosomes. Since these adhesive devices appear to have a more complex three-dimensional organization they are referred to as 'fasciae adherentes' instead of maculae adherentes (= desmosome). The actin filaments of the I-bands above and below appear to insert into these densities (for details see Fig. 189). The cross-banded pattern of the myofibrils is almost identical to that of skeletal muscle (cf. Fig. 195). Arrowhead (►) points to a small portion of the tubular network of the sarcoplasmic reticulum. Magnification 30,000 ×.

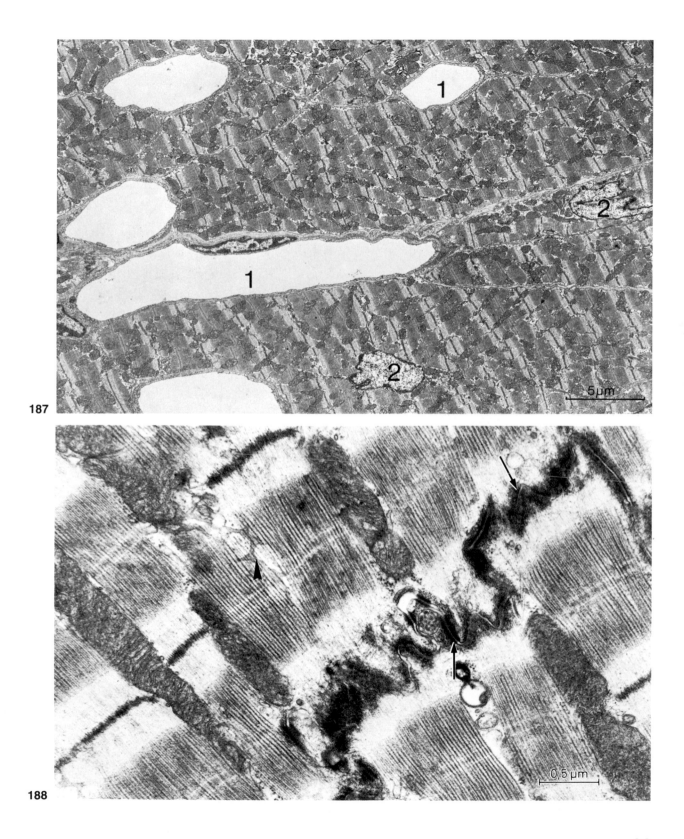

187

188

Cardiac muscle – Electron microscopy

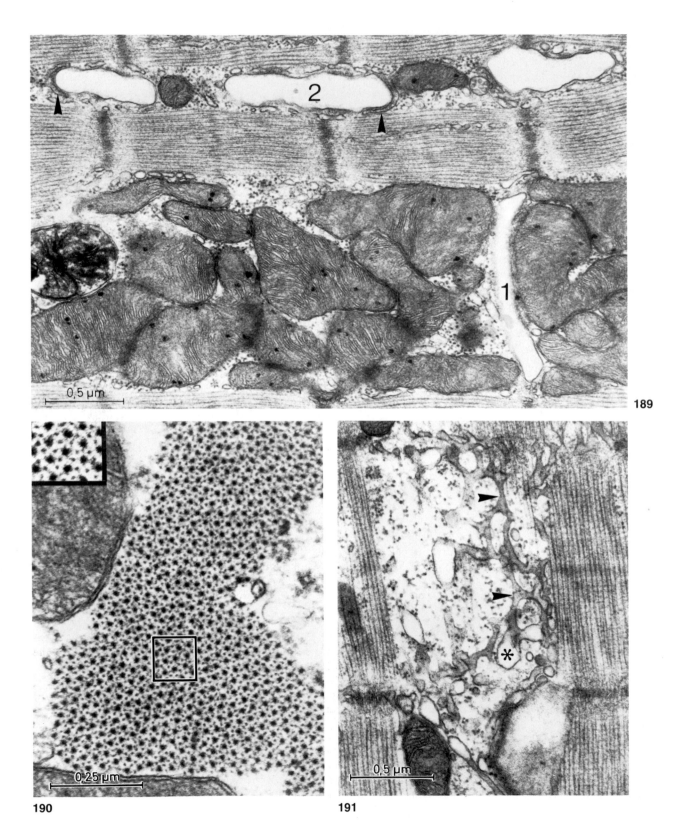

189

190

191

90

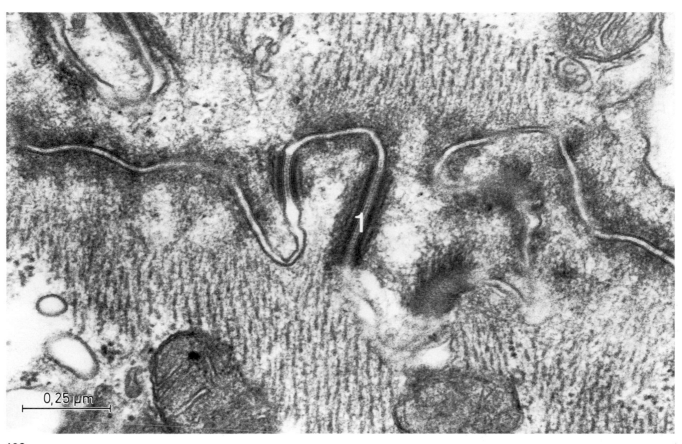

0,25 µm

192

Fig. 189. Part of a longitudinally sectioned cardiac cell to illustrate cytologic details like cross-banded pattern of myofibrils and large number of tightly packed interfibrillar mitochondria with elaborate cristae (from guinea pig papillary muscle). In this species (guinea pig) the transverse tubules (**1**) are not only extremely wide, but they also course parallel (**2**) to the long axis of the myofibrils. They also make close contact with the sarcoplasmic reticulum which appears at these sites as slit-like membrane-bound cavities (►), known as subsarcolemmal cisternae. Magnification 40,000 ×.

Fig. 190. High-power electron micrograph of a cross-sectioned cardiac myofibril at the A-band level to illustrate regular pattern of thin and thick filaments. Each myosin filament is surrounded by six actin filaments resulting in a very precise hexagonal array of the thick filaments (boxed area and inset). From guinea pig papillary muscle. Magnification 96,000 × and 164,000 ×, respectively.

Fig. 191. Longitudinal section of a cardiac cell from guinea pig papillary muscle favorably cut through sarcoplasmic reticulum (►) so that at least parts of this tubular network can be recognized as a continuum. Asterisk marks irregular focal dilatation of the sarcoplasmic reticulum. Magnification 44,000 ×.

Fig. 192. High-power electron micrograph (primary magnification 40,000 ×) of a segment of an intercalated disk from guinea pig papillary muscle. The adjoining cardiac cells display elaborate interdigitations with each other, giving rise to a complex wavy course of their sarcolemmata, which reveal characteristic desmosomes (**1**). The latter are just one representative of the variant adhesive devices occurring along the length of the intercalated disks. Magnification 92,000 ×.

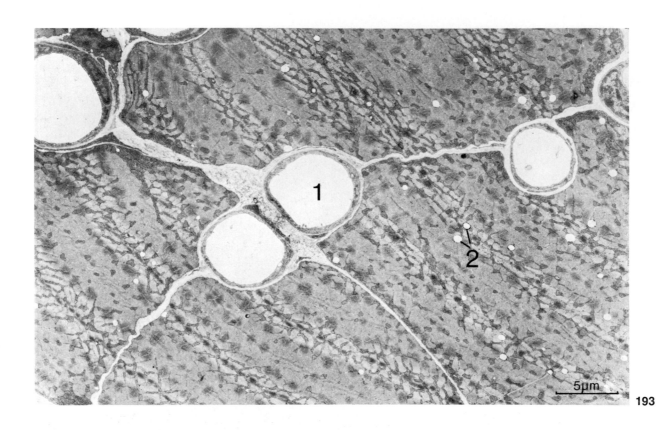

193

Fig. 193.   Cross-sectioned skeletal muscle fibers from the tongue of a cat. A rough estimate of the size difference between skeletal muscle fibers and smooth or cardiac muscle cells can be gained by a comparison of this micrograph with Figure 186, showing that the same area that contains only parts of four muscle fibers encloses at least seven whole cardiac cells. **1** Capillary lumen;   **2** Lipid vacuoles.   Magnification 3,000 ×.

Fig. 194.   Longitudinal section of skeletal muscle fibers from the same specimen and shown with the same magnification as in the preceding electron micrograph. In this case it is a "white" fiber because of the low number of subsarcolemmal and interfibrillar mitochondria (→). As the prominent Z-Lines are flanked by very narrow I-bands, the fiber is almost completely contracted. **1** Capillary lumen;   **2** Lipid vacuoles;   **3** Lumen of arteriole;   **4** Nucleus of a muscle fiber.   Magnification 3,000 ×.

Fig. 195.   Higher-power electron micrograph of longitudinally sectioned myofibrils from Syrian hamster cutaneous muscle (panniculus carnosus). The upper myofibrils ([) display the full length of one sarcomere (= distance between two successive Z-lines: ⊢——⊣) with all the main transverse bands. The I-bands (I) consist only of thin (actin) filaments, which extend from the Z-line through the I-band and into the A-band (A). The major component of the A-band are the thick, 1.5 μm long myosin filaments, which are limited to the A-band. The latter is subdivided into an H-band bisected by the centrally placed M-line. The H-band corresponds to that segment of the A-band into which the actin filaments do not reach and is, therefore, dependent upon the state of contraction. The M-band is due to delicate filamentous cross-bridges between the myosin filaments. Near the A-I-junctions are triads (encircled) that consist of minute T-tubules flanked by larger vacuoles, the cross-sectioned terminal cisternae of the sarcoplasmic reticulum. Inset: Single triad in longitudinal section. The membranes of both cisternae (★) facing the narrow T-tubule appear scalloped.   Magnification 27,000 × and 50,000 ×, respectively.

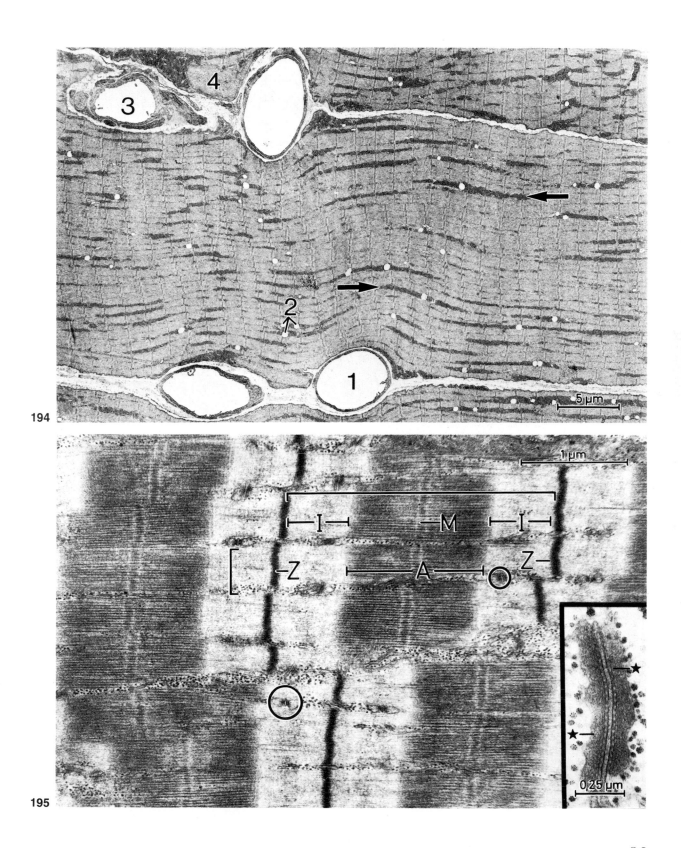

194

195

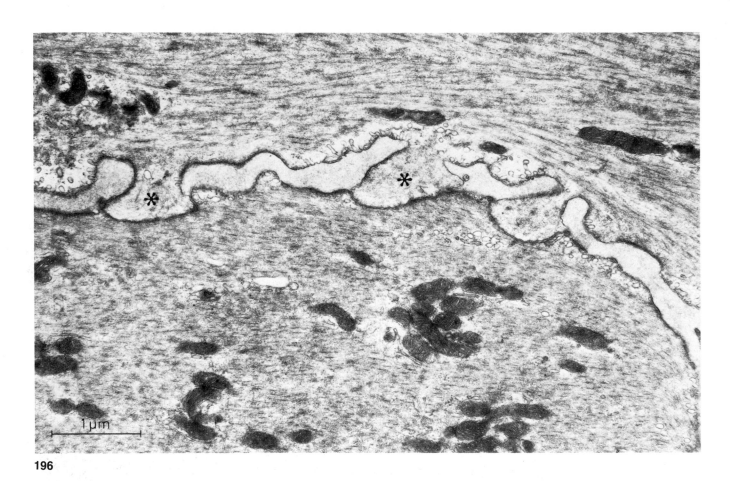

196

Fig. 196. Smooth muscle cells found in the muscular tunic of a wide variety of hollow organs establish close contacts with each other by projecting variously shaped, often foot-like expansions (✳) towards the adjoining cells. These processes frequently fit into corresponding grooves or pits with the opposed membranes being not more than 15–20 nm apart and often revealing gap-junctions known in this location as 'nexus'. These are, therefore, the sites for intramural transmission of electrical stimuli. From rat portal vein. Magnification 23,000×.

Fig. 197. The finer ramifications of the impulse conducting system of the heart are the Purkinje fibers, a highly specialized type of cardiac muscle cells (from guinea pig papillary muscle). These plumpish elements stand out clearly in electron micrographs due to their large electron lucent cell bodies (**1**) containing a significantly reduced number of myofibrils, which are displaced towards the periphery (**2**). **3** Ordinary cardiomyocytes; **4** Erythrocyte within a capillary. Magnification 5,000×.

Fig. 198. The transmission of the motor nerve impulse to the muscle fiber occurs at highly specialized sites, the neuromuscular junctions or motor end plates. They consist of terminal axon swellings (**1**) containing numerous electron lucent (synaptic) vesicles together with mitochondria. These axon terminals lie in a shallow synaptic trough formed by the surface of the muscle fiber. The sarcolemma lining this groove is pleated into numerous branching folds (**2**) into which the external or basal lamina projects filling the synaptic cleft (►) which separates the axon terminal from the muscle fiber. Magnification 11,000×.

94

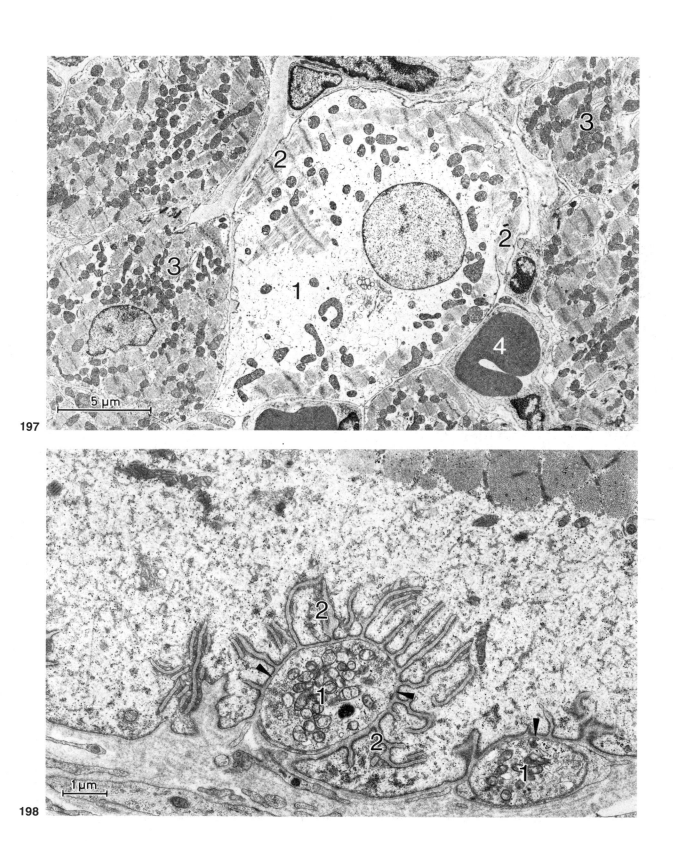

197

198

Glial cell nuclei

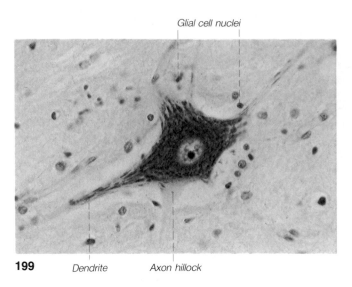

199   Dendrite   Axon hillock

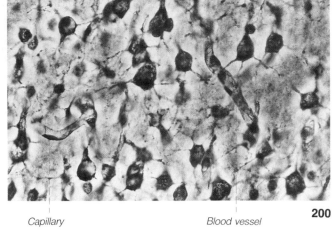

Capillary   Blood vessel   **200**

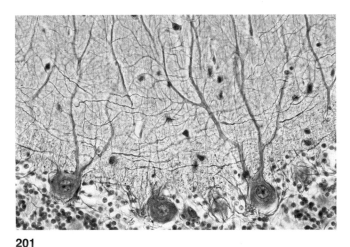

201

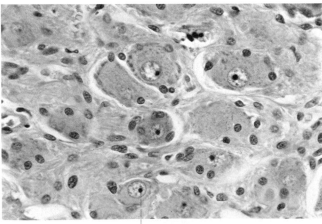

202   Nucleus with nucleolus

Fig. 199. Multipolar nerve cell from the anterior horn of the canine spinal cord showing several dendrites that can be identified by the presence of Nissl bodies in their proximal parts. The axon and that part of the cell body from which it emerges, the axon hillock, are notably free of Nissl substance. The strongly basophilic clumps of material are called Nissl substance after their discoverer and they are the light microscopic equivalent of a well-developed rough ER. Note the large spherical nucleus with its prominent nucleolus. Toluidine blue staining. Magnification 380×.

Fig. 200. Multipolar nerve cells from monkey brain cortex illustrated by a silver impregnation technique. Short spine-like processes originate abruptly and radiate from the prominent nucleated cell bodies. A distinction between dendrites and neurites is not possible in this preparation. Notice the remarkable diversity in size of the nerve cells shown with the same magnification in Figures 199, 200 and 202. Staining: Cajal's method. Magnification 380×.

Fig. 201. The fan-shaped dendritic arborization of a Purkinje cell from rat cerebellar cortex. The axon is given off from the end of the flask-like cell bodies opposite the dendrites. Silver impregnation (Bodian). Magnification 240×.

Fig. 202. Multipolar nerve cells in an autonomic ganglion found in a human adrenal medulla. Most of these cells are spherical or ovoid and their large vesicular nuclei and prominent nucleoli allow for easy identification. Mallory-azan staining. Magnification 380×.

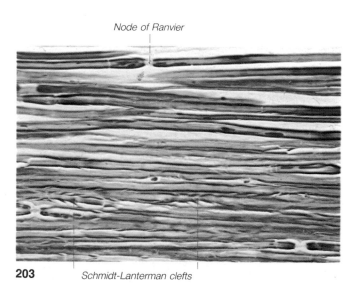

Node of Ranvier

203   *Schmidt-Lanterman clefts*

Fig. 203. Longitudinal section of rabbit sciatic nerve fixed in OsO_4 to preserve and blacken the myelin. Nodes of Ranvier (= interruptions of the myelin sheath) can be see in both the upper and lower parts of the micrograph. The funnel-shaped notches (= clefts of Schmidt-Lanterman) are focal areas where the myelin lamellae are separated by Schwann cell cytoplasm, but retain their continuity. Fixation in OsO_4, no counterstain. Magnification 240×.

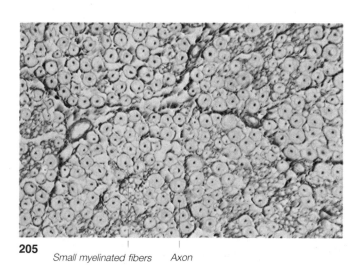

204

Fig. 204. Feline spinal nerve, the fibers shown in both cross- and longitudinal section. When cross-sectioned, the myelin sheaths appear as dark-brown rings around an unstained central core, the axon. Fixation in OsO_4, no counterstain. Magnification 150×.

Fig. 205. Cross-section of a myelinated peripheral nerve (human sciatic nerve). Compare with Figure 207. The shrunken axons appear as dark-violet or black spots surrounded by the faint yellow myelin sheath. Interspersed between these thick myelinated fibers are groups of small nerve fibers, either poor in or devoid of myelin (= non-myelinated fibers). The Schwann cell nuclei are not visible as no counterstaining was performed. Picric acid and indigocarmine staining. Magnification 240×.

205   *Small myelinated fibers*   *Axon*

Schwann cell nuclei

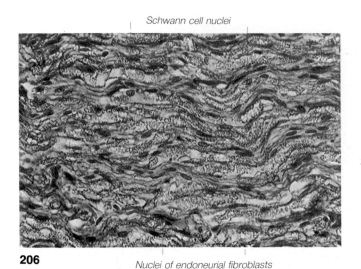

206

Nuclei of endoneurial fibroblasts

Fig. 206. Longitudinal section through a dorsal root from a human spinal cord. During routine histologic preparation much of the myelin sheath is dissolved as a result of the use of lipid solvents, leaving behind a proteinaceous residue called neurokeratin. The large elliptical nuclei are those of Schwann cells, while the elongated ones belong to fibroblasts in the endoneurium. Mallory-azan staining. Magnification 240 ×.

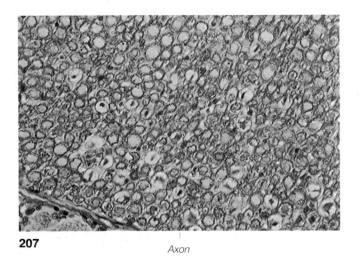

207

Axon

Fig. 207. Cross-section through a feline spinal nerve, the variably sized axons of which show a finely granulated appearance (= neurokeratin) of their myelin sheaths following lipid extraction (see also Fig. 206). Here and there the axis cylinders are condensed into a central deeply red-staining mass. Mallory-azan staining. Magnification 240 ×.

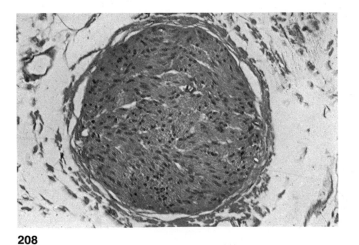

208

Fig. 208. Cross-section through a small non-myelinated nerve from the vascular bundle of human spleen. In this specimen note that subdivisions by connective tissue septa are lacking and that the axons are cut in all planes of section because of their twisting course. Another characteristic of non-myelinated nerves is the large number of cells, here revealed by their nuclei. H&E staining. Magnification 240 ×.

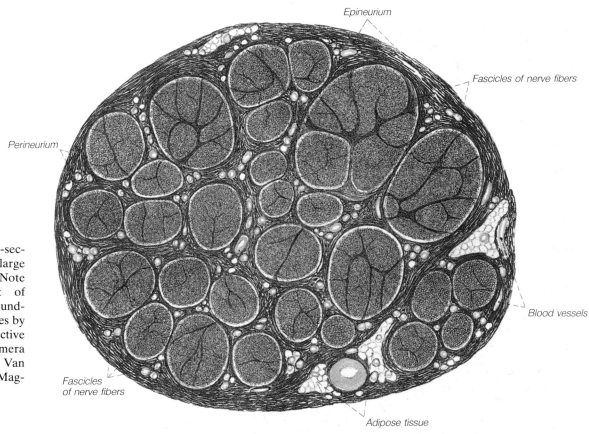

Epineurium

Fascicles of nerve fibers

Perineurium

Blood vessels

Fascicles of nerve fibers

Adipose tissue

Fig. 209. Cross-section trough a large peripheral nerve. Note the arrangement of nerve fibers into bundles of different sizes by means of connective tissue septa (camera lucida drawing). Van Gieson staining. Magnification 35 ×.

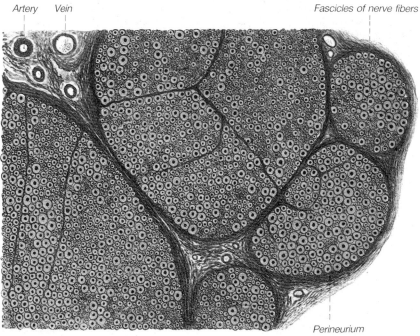

Artery   Vein

Fascicles of nerve fibers

Perineurium

Fig. 210. A higher magnification of several nerve fiber bundles reveals the individual axons as distinct circular profiles of varying diameter. The axis cylinders are clearly demarcated from their surrounding myelin sheaths by their different staining properties (camera lucida drawing). Van Gieson staining. Magnification 150 ×.

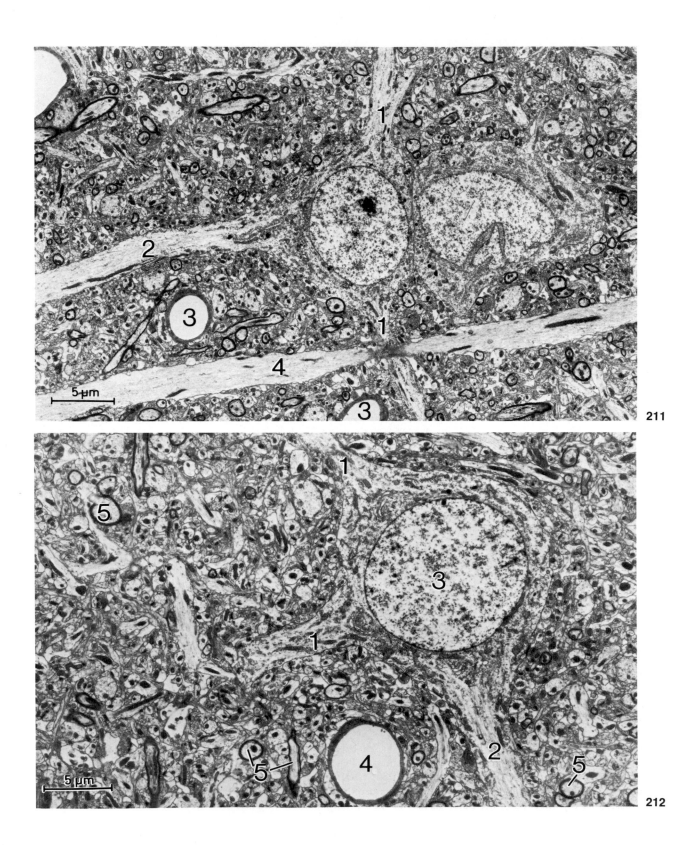

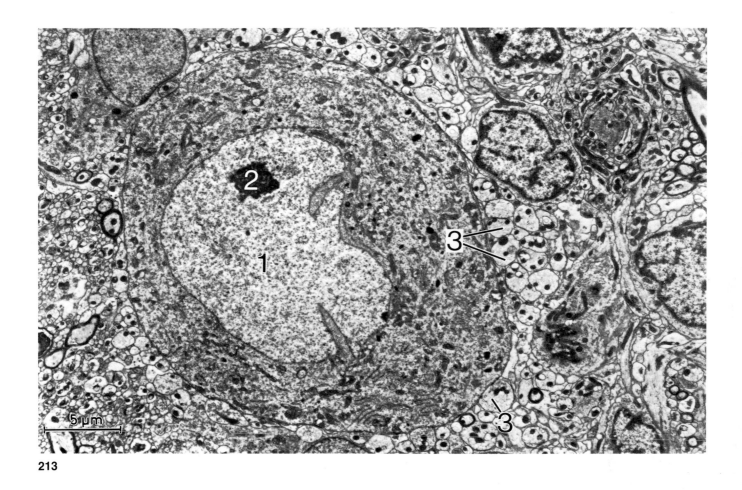

213

Low-power electron micrographs from rat cerebral cortex to illustrate the fine structural appearance of the various components of the central nervous tissue.

Fig. 211.   Two closely apposed nerve cells the left one of which clearly displays several processes radiating from the cell body, thereby disclosing its multipolar nature. The processes projecting up- and downward are dendrites (**1**), whereas the one coursing horizontally represents the axon (**2**). It usually has a larger diameter and is more electron-lucent than the dendrites due to the absence of rough ER. **3** Lumina of capillaries; **4** Another axon crossed by the downward dendrite. Magnification 3,500×.

Fig. 212.   Single multipolar nerve cell showing three of its processes two of which definitely represent dendrites (**1**) whereas the third (**2**), probably the axon, cannot be classified with absolute certainty. The large vesicular nucleus (**3**) has a diameter almost three times that of a nearby capillary (**4**). The surrounding neuropil is dominated by cross-sectioned cell processes of all kinds, quite a number of which are axons enwrapped by a myelin sheath of moderate thickness (**5**). Magnification 3,500×.

Fig. 213.   Pear-shaped cell body (soma) of a Purkinje cell from rat cerebellar cortex shown with the same magnification as the two preceding electron micrographs to allow an immediate comparison of these three nerve cells. In this case the nucleus (**1**) is almost as large as the entire soma of the nerve cells depicted in the other two electron micrographs. The nucleus contains a prominent nucleolus (**2**) and a karyolymph consisting mainly of euchromatin. Note also the numerous electron-lucent cytoplasmic profiles (**3**), mostly dendritic processes, closely attached to the outer surface of the Purkinje soma. Magnification 4,000×.

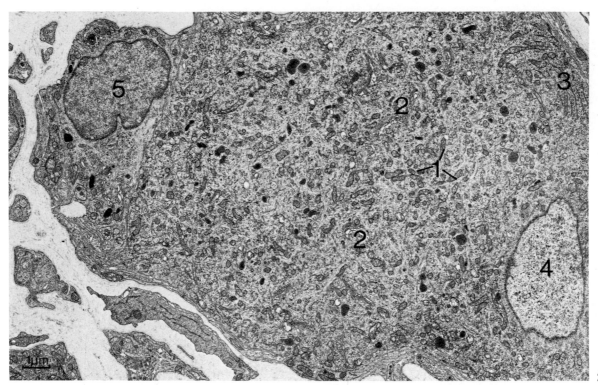

214

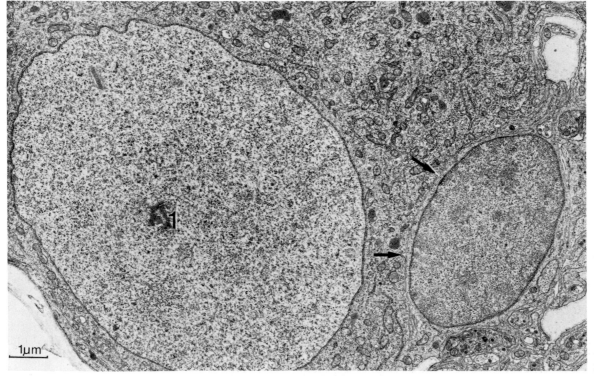

215

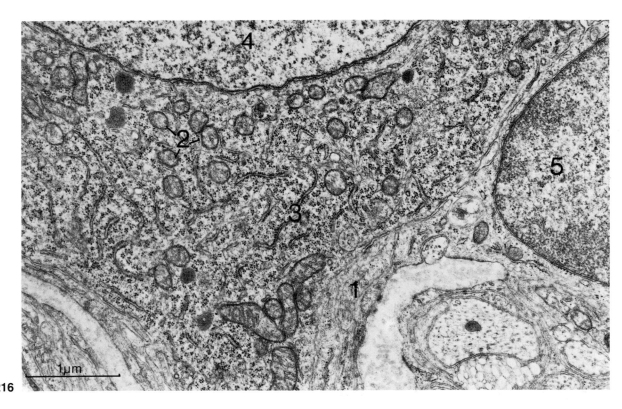

Fig. 216. Peripheral part of an autonomic ganglion cell (same specimen as in the preceding two figures), showing the origin of a dendrite with a satellite cell process (**1**) closely attached to its surface. The nerve cell cytoplasm contains numerous mitochondria (**2**), many cisternae of a well-developed rough ER (**3**) and large numbers of free ribosomes. **4** Nucleus of the nerve cell; **5** Nucleus of the satellite cell. Magnification 24,500×.

Fig. 214. Low-power view of a nerve cell in an autonomic ganglion from the pancreas of a cat. The perikaryon contains many small mitochondria (**1**), several Golgi complexes (**2**) and a well-developed rough ER that in places forms regular stacks of parallel cisternae (**3**). Only a small portion of the peripherally placed nucleus (**4**) is visible in this micrograph. **5** Nucleus of a satellite cell. Magnification 7,000×.

Fig. 215. Another neuron from the same ganglion illustrates the large vesicular nucleus (**1**) together with its nucleolus and the extremely narrow space (→) intervening between nerve and satellite cell. Magnification 10,000×.

Nerve fibers, myelinated – Electron microscopy

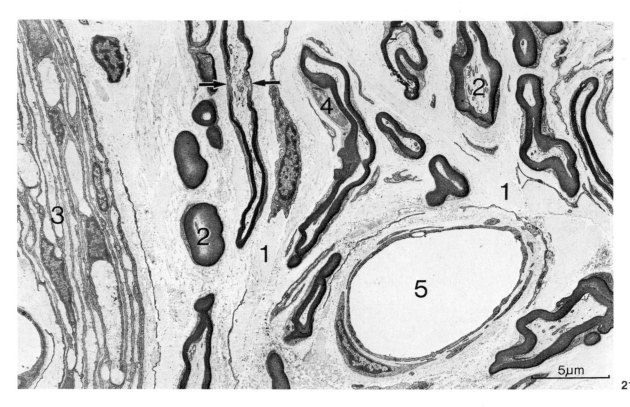

Fig. 217. Peripheral parts of a myelinated rabbit nerve with axons (**2**) cut in various planes of section and loosely arranged in abundant connective tissue (**1** collagen fibrils). The nerve is shielded from its environment by a multilayered cellular sheath (**3**) composed of fibroblasts and their processes. The arrows point to a node of Ranvier. **4** Nucleus of Schwann cell; **5** Postcapillary venule. Magnification 4,500 ×.

Fig. 218. Longitudinal section through a rabbit axon with myelin sheath (**1**) and (**2**) sheath of Schwann (= neurilemmal sheath). Note the bundle of filaments (**3**) in the cytoplasm of an adjacent fibroblast. **4** Mitochondrion. Magnification 30,000 ×.

Fig. 219. a) Close-up of the preceding micrograph disclosing the characteristic layered appearance of the myelin sheath with periodicity of 12 nm. The inner aspect of the myelin sheath is separated from the axoplasm (**2**) by the axolemma (**1**), while its outer surface is covered by the Schwann cell (**3**). Magnification 80,000 ×.
b) Longitudinal section through an unmyelinated nerve fiber with prominent neurofilaments (**1**) and neurotubules (**2**). Compare with Figure 222. Magnification 54,000 ×.

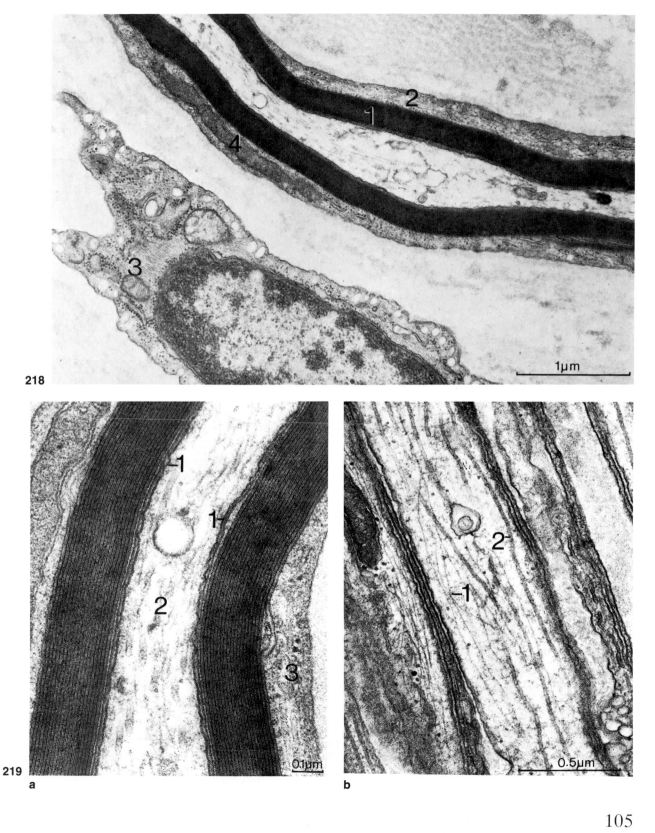

218

1µm

219

a

0.1µm

b

0.5µm

Nerve fibers, unmyelinated – Electron microscopy

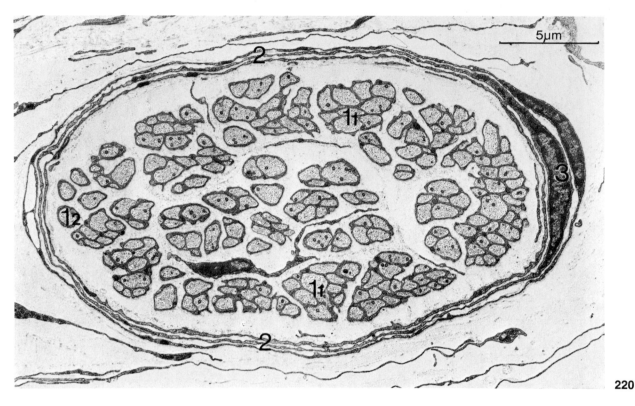

220

Fig. 220. Cross-section through a non-myelinated autonomic nerve (rat) completely enclosed and thus separated from the surrounding connective tissue by a multilayered sheath (**2**), the perithelium or perineural "epithelium", composed of fibroblasts and their veil-like cytoplasmic processes. The darker-staining cytoplasm of Schwann cells encloses the more translucent axons either in groups ($\mathbf{1}_1$) of varying size and number or individually ($\mathbf{1}_2$). At this low magnification the axons have a finely speckled appearance. **3** Nucleus of a fibroblast. Magnification 5,000 ×.

Fig. 221. Part of a similar autonomic nerve to the one in the preceding micrograph showing either one ($\mathbf{1}_2$) or several ($\mathbf{1}_1$) axons wrapped in an often complex fashion (→) by the thin cytoplasmic lamellae of a Schwann cell. **2** Mitochondria. Magnification 24,000 ×.

Fig. 222. High-power micrograph of two axons from the preceding figure showing bundles of loosely associated filaments (**1**) and coarser microtubules (**2**). Although these structures are separate entities, together they form the submicroscopic material that is visualized as neurofibrils in light microscopic preparations after silver impregnation techniques. Note that the free edges (✳) of the delicate Schwann cell lamellae overlap each other over a considerable distance. Magnification 53,000 ×.

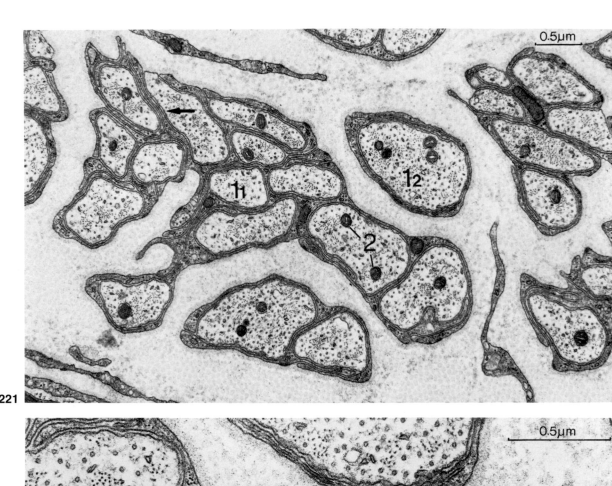

221

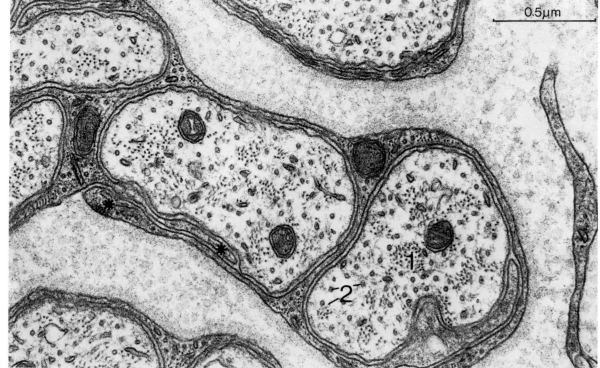

222

Nervous tissue – Neuroglia

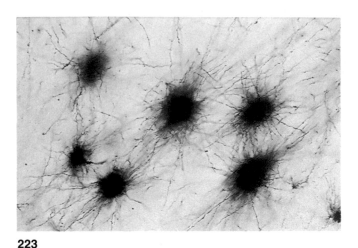

223

The demonstration of the various types of glial cells in the central nervous system is possible only with the use of special, often rather complicated staining procedures.
In many histological courses only a restricted number of such precious preparations is therefore available.
(The specimens for Figures 223, 224, 227 and 228 were kindly supplied by Prof. Dr. G. Kersting, Bonn, FRG).

Oligodendrocyte

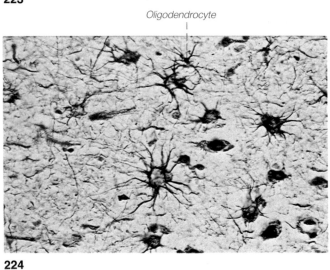

224

Fig. 223. Fibrous astrocytes from human cerebral white matter as seen with the Golgi method. The large number of silver granules accumulated on the cell surfaces cause an apparent enlargement of the cell and even obscure the nucleus. Still visible, however, are the many long occasionally branched processes projecting in all directions from the perikarya and responsible for the term "fibrous". Staining: Golgi's chrome silver method. Magnification 240×.

Fig. 224. Several astrocytes from human cerebral gray matter with short highly branched processes attached to the large cell bodies, the "protoplasmic astrocytes". In the upper part of the micrograph is a smaller oligodendrocyte with fewer more delicate processes. Staining: Bielschowsky's method. Magnification 380×.

- - - *Astrocytes* - - -

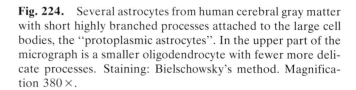

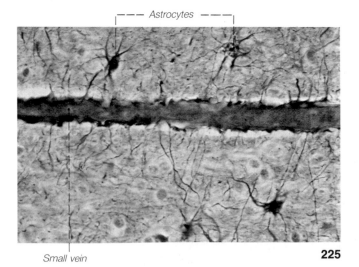

Small vein

225

Fig. 225. Fibrous astrocytes from human cerebral cortex forming a perivascular glial sheath by surrounding the smallest blood vessels with the foot-like expansions of their processes. Staining: Held's method. Magnification 380×.

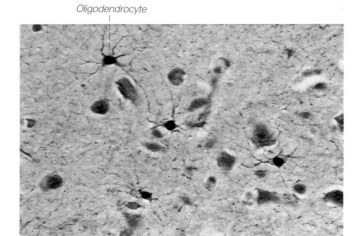

Astrocytic cell body

226

Capillary   Astrocytic process

Fig. 226. Higher magnification clearly reveals the extension of a fibrous astrocyte closely attached to a capillary (human cerebral cortex). Staining: Held's method. Magnification 960×.

Oligodendrocyte

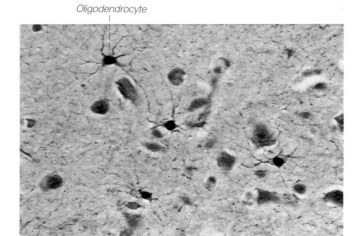

227

Fig. 227. Oligodendrocytes from human cerebral cortex. The whole cell body is smaller than that of an astrocyte and hence is nearly completely filled by the nucleus, as is also the case in lymphocytes. Since only the nucleus is thus seen in routine preparations, oligodendrocytes can be difficult to identify. They are frequently found immediately adjacent to nerve cell bodies, as here, and then classified as satellite or perineural cells. Staining: Cajal's method. Magnification 380×.

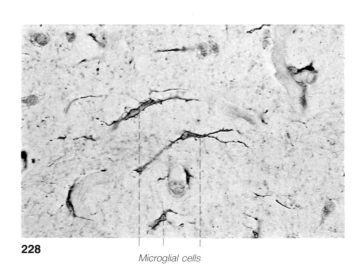

228

Microglial cells

Fig. 228. Microglial cells from human cerebral cortex. These cells are small and give off only a few delicate and tortuous processes with spines. They are believed to be capable of ameboid movements and phagocytosis and therefore play a role in the removal of cellular debris in a variety of pathological conditions, e.g., following an apoplectic stroke. Staining: Hortega's method. Magnification 380×.

Microscopic Anatomy

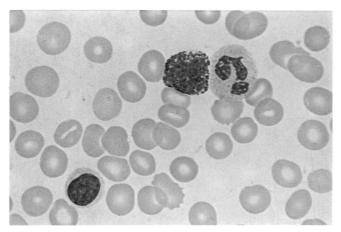

229

One of the most common routine tests used in clinical medicine is the differential blood count, i.e., the determination of the percentages of the various types of white blood cells (leukocytes) in dried blood smears by means of the varying structural and staining properties of the cells. Because the special staining procedures depend on skilled and experienced technical assistance, one is often confronted with poor quality in such preparations.

May-Grünwald staining has been used throughout in Figures 229–235.

Fig. 229. Three different types of leukocytes. In the upper part of the micrograph there is a cell filled with large basophilic granules (= basophilic granulocyte or "basophil") lying beside a neutrophilic polymorphonuclear leukocyte. At the lower left is a lymphocyte with its characteristic high nucleocytoplasmic ratio (large nucleus surrounded by a thin rim of cytoplasm). Note the size differences of the leukocyte types and compare them with the erythrocytes – size is one of the criteria essential for correct classification. Magnification 960×.

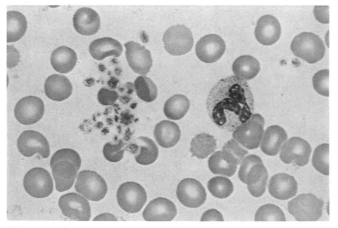

230

Fig. 230. Among the erythrocytes a cluster of blood platelets (= thrombocytes) can be seen. Platelet detail is not visible at this magnification. To the right is a neutrophilic granulocyte (= "polymorph" or "neutrophil") with a moderately lobed nucleus and numerous fine granules that are shown by eletron microscopy to be small pleomorphic lysosomes (cf. Fig. 237). Magnification 960×.

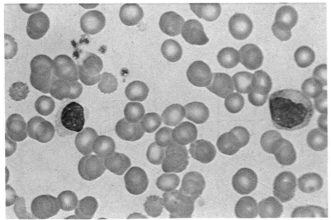

231

Fig. 231. Toward the left side of this micrograph is a "large" lymphocyte, while a monocyte characterized by its large indented and often bean-shaped nucleus lies at the right side. Several platelets are visible in the upper left corner. Magnification 750×.

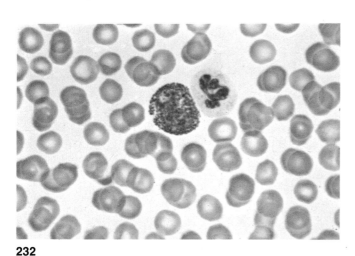

232

Drumstick

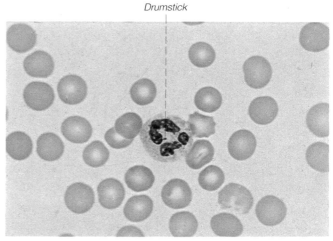

233

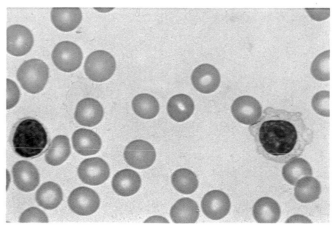

234

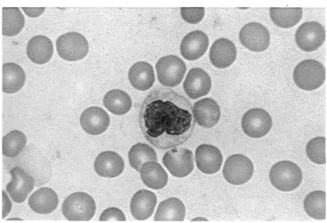

235

Fig. 232. The central large cell is an eosinophilic granulocyte with a bilobed nucleus, which is one of the characteristics of this type of leukocyte. Even if the granules are not stained as distinctly as in this example, their size and number allow for their identification (cf. Fig. 230). Electron microscopy shows that the granules (= lysosomes) have a banded appearance with a prominent central crystal lattice (see Fig. 238). The white blood cell adjacent to the "eosinophil" is a neutrophilic granulocyte. Magnification 960×.

Fig. 233. Neutrophilic granulocyte with a lobed nucleus showing a "drumstick" on its upper segment. This nuclear appendage represents the sex chromatin and is found in 1 in every 36 neutrophils in women. Because this ratio varies and since drumsticks are found even in normal male neutrophils (maximum 1 in 1000), 2,000 neutrophils must be examined in such a leukocyte test to allow for an exact chromosomal sex identification. Magnification 960×.

Fig. 234. This micrograph contains a small (left) and large (right) lymphocyte clearly differentiated by their different nucleocytoplasmic ratios. Small lymphocytes have only a thin rim of cytoplasm that is often difficult to see, while the more abundant pale cytoplasm of larger but younger lymphocytes displays tiny azurophilic granules. Magnification 960×.

Fig. 235. Monocyte with a large indented nucleus. Fine azurophilic granules are present in the faintly staining basophilic cytoplasm. Although the nuclei of monocytes are not always bean-shaped, they never have the circular outlines seen regularly in "large" lymphocytes. Magnification 960×.

113

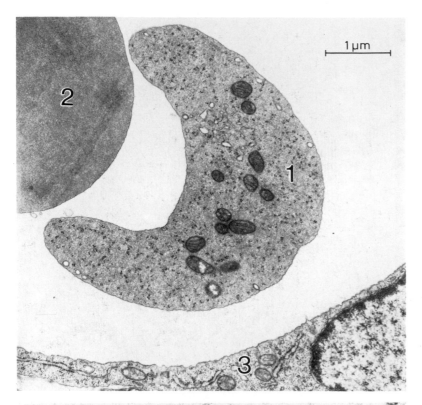

Fig. 236. Freshly produced erythrocyte (**1**) lying close to a mature red blood cell (**2**) in a newly formed capillary from Syrian hamster subcutaneous tissue. Such reticulocytes still contain several mitochondria together with ribosomes which give rise to a supravitally stainable fine granular network (cf. Fig. 247). **3** Endothelial cell. Magnification 17,000×.

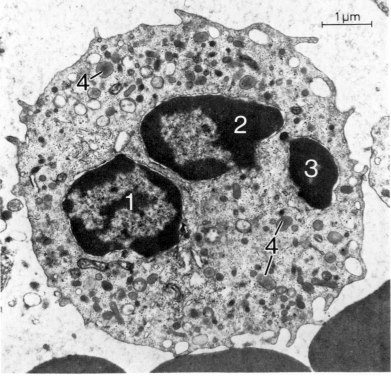

Fig. 237. Mature human polymorphonuclear neutrophil. Several lobes of the nucleus (**1–3**) are present together with numerous granules varying in size and shape. The latge variety (**4**) corresponds to the azurophilic granules seen with the light microscope, but all of these granules represent lysosomes. Magnification 13,000×.

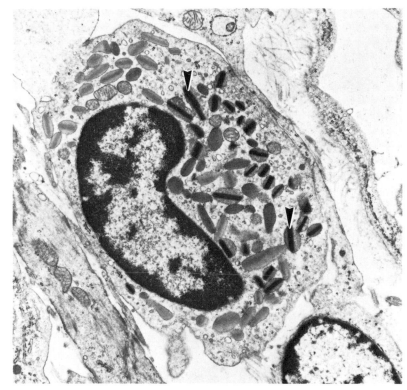

Fig. 238. Mature eosinophil from rat intestinal mucosa. These cells are characterized by the large size and by the shape of their specific granules which in addition contain a central discoid crystal (▶). As in neutrophils these granules represent lysosomes. Magnification 14,000 ×.

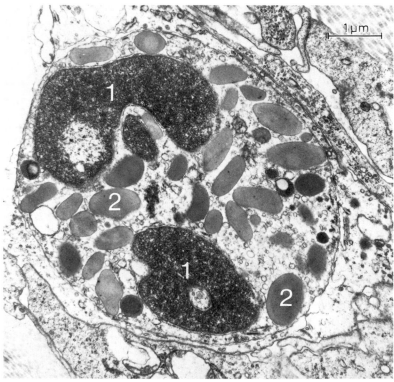

Fig. 239. Mature basophil from Syrian hamster subcutaneous tissue showing two nuclear lobes (**1**) and numerous specific granules (**2**). They are distinctly membrane-bound and display homogeneous contents varying in electron opacity. Compared to the preceding eosinophilic granules the basophilics are significantly larger (both figures are of the same final magnification), and they contain heparin, histamine, and, in rodents, serotonin. Magnification 14,000 ×.

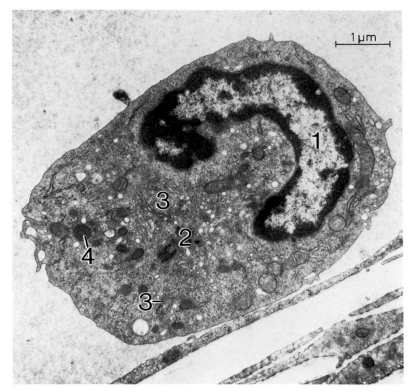

Fig. 240. Intravascular monocyte lying close to the endothelium of a larger mucosal vein from guinea pig gallbladder. The nucleus (**1**) shows its characteristic horseshoe shape, and the cytoplasm displays a prominent centrosphere (**2**), several Golgi complexes (**3**), and some electron dense granules (**4**) of lysosomal nature. They all represent typical structural features of monocytes at the level of electron microscopy. Magnification 14,000×.

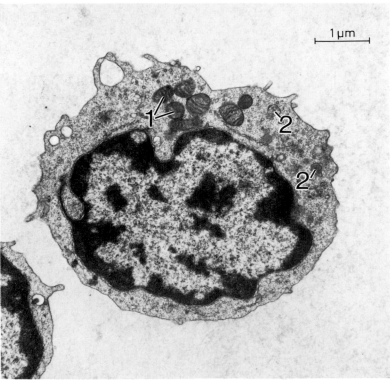

Fig. 241. Intravascular mediumsized lymphocyte from rabbit respiratory mucosa showing the nucleocytoplasmic relationship, typically very much in favor of the nucleus. The cytoplasm contains several mitochondria (**1**) and a few lysosomes (**2**). Magnification 14,000×.

Fig. 242. An intravascular aggregate of thrombocytes in a larger vein from Syrian hamster cheek pouch. The moderately dense cytoplasm contains several rather large membrane-bound granules (✳) of almost identical electron opacity. A second type of granules, known as dense bodies, shows an extremely electron dense material (►) often separated by a lucent space from the surrounding membrane and contains serotonin. A third type of membrane-bound cavities corresponds to tubular invaginations of the cell membrane and is known as "canaliculi". The total mass of granules, mitochondria and other formed components constitute the stainable center of a platelet called "granulomere" in light microscopy. This is surrounded by the outer homogeneous "hyalomere". **1** Nucleus of endothelial cell; **2** Nucleus of smooth muscle cell. Magnification 17,000 ×.

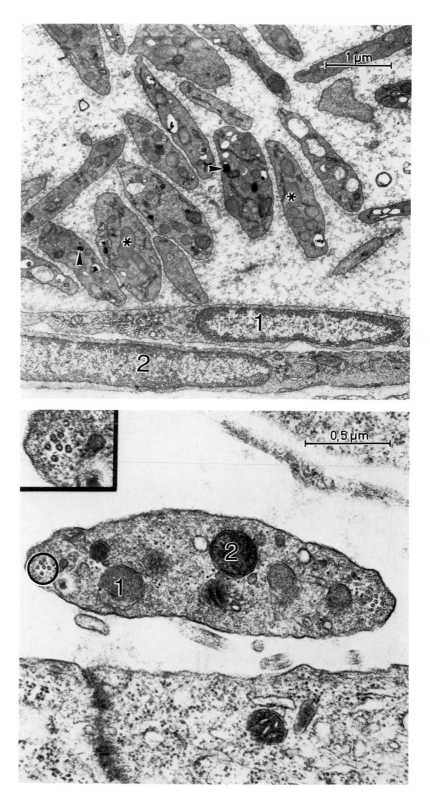

Fig. 243. Thrombocyte at higher magnification (44,000 ×) to illustrate cytoplasmic components to better advantage. Notice the distinct bundle of cross sectioned microtubules (circled) running circumferentially around the periphery of platelets and serving as a cytoskeleton.
1 Granule; **2** Mitochondrion. Inset illustrates circled area at a magnification of 66,000 ×.

117

Red bone marrow and reticulocytes

Adipose cell

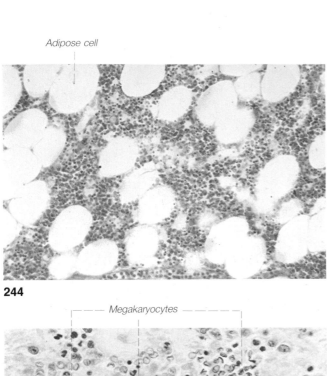

244

Megakaryocytes

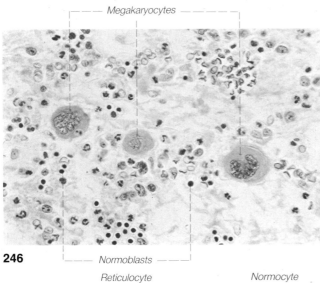

246

Normoblasts

Reticulocyte   Normocyte

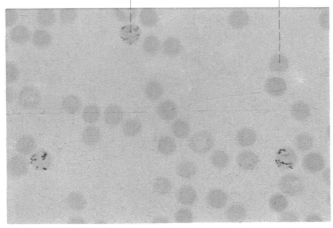

247

Normoblasts

245

Fig. 244. Red hemopoietic bone marrow (section through the spongiosa of a juvenile femoral diaphysis); osseous trabeculae not included in this micrograph. Numerous fat cells are interspersed between the cellular strands which consist of reticular connective tissue packed with innumerable cells belonging to the various stages of erythro- and granulopoiesis. H & E staining. Magnification 95 ×.

Fig. 245. A higher magnification of the same specimen shown in the preceding micrograph reveals various components of erythro- and granulopoiesis. Only normoblasts, identified by their dense round nuclei, are clearly defined. H & E staining. Magnification 600 ×.

Fig. 246. Three megakaryocytes from human bone marrow. These cells are characterized by their large size and by their apparent multinuclear nature, the latter due to the varying and complex arrangement of the many nuclear lobes. Platelet originate from these cells by fragmentation from the megakaryocytic pseudopodia. The dense round nuclei in this specimen belong to normoblasts. H & E staining. Magnification 380 ×.

Fig. 247. Reticulocytes [do not confuse this term with reticular (reticulum) cells] from the peripheral blood. The supravital staining with brilliant cresyl blue, performed by mixing the stain with fresh blood prior to making the smear, reveals a fine granular network in these immature erythrocytes due to the precipitation and aggregation of ribosomes caused by the dye. An increase in reticulocytes (normally 1−2% of the erythrocytes) in the peripheral blood is an index of an increased rate of red cell formation by the bone marrow, e.g., following severe hemorrhage. Supravital staining with brilliant cresyl blue. Magnification 960 ×.

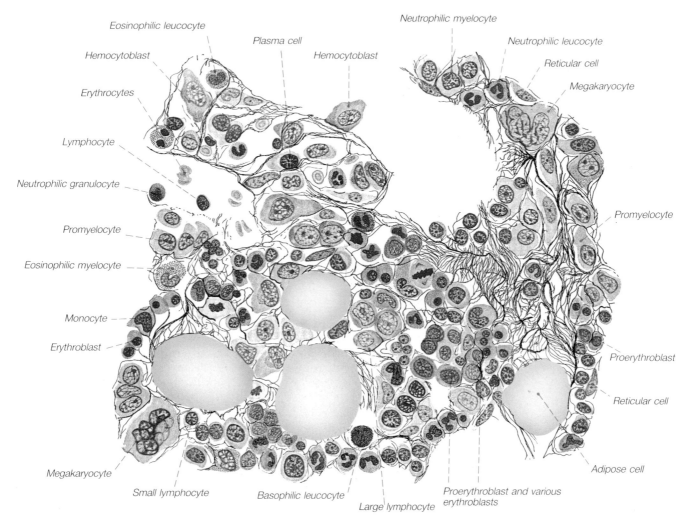

Eosinophilic leucocyte

Hemocytoblast

Erythrocytes

Lymphocyte

Neutrophilic granulocyte

Promyelocyte

Eosinophilic myelocyte

Monocyte

Erythroblast

Megakaryocyte

Small lymphocyte

Basophilic leucocyte

Large lymphocyte

Plasma cell

Hemocytoblast

Neutrophilic myelocyte

Neutrophilic leucocyte

Reticular cell

Megakaryocyte

Promyelocyte

Proerythroblast

Reticular cell

Adipose cell

Proerythroblast and various erythroblasts

Fig. 248. Partly schematic drawing of human bone marrow and its supporting network of reticular fibers (from Patzelt: *Histologie*, 3rd ed., Urban & Schwarzenberg, Vienna 1948). Staining: H & E combined with silver impregnation. Magnification approximately 1200 ×.

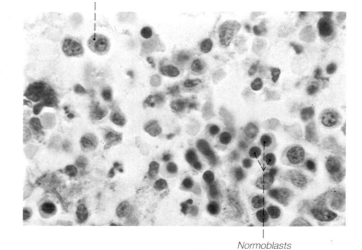

Eosinophilic myelocyte

Normoblasts

249. Micrograph of human bone marrow for comparison with the preceding drawing. Although most of the cell types are not identifiable, normoblasts stand out because of their dense round nuclei, myelocytes because of their specific granules. Giemsa staining. Magnification 960 ×.

Lymphoid organs – Tonsils

The lymphoid organs can be divided into lymphoreticular and lymphoepithelial organs. The main lymphoepithelial organs are the three tonsils, each of which is a combination of an epithelial surface and a supporting lymphoid tissue. Identification of the tonsils depends on 1) the different epithelia (only the pharyngeal tonsil has a respiratory epithelium, 2) the size, since sections usually contain the whole organ (the palatine tonsil is much larger than the other two), and 3) the composition of the surrounding tissue (only the lingual tonsil is associated with large amounts of glandular tissue).

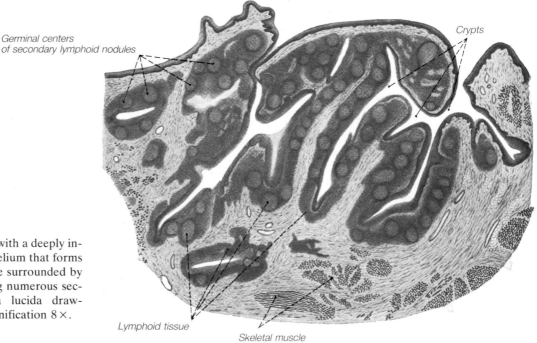

Germinal centers of secondary lymphoid nodules

Crypts

Lymphoid tissue

Skeletal muscle

Fig. 250. Palatine tonsil with a deeply invaginating squamous epthelium that forms branching crypts which are surrounded by lymphoid tissue containing numerous secondary nodules (camera lucida drawing). H&E staining. Magnification 8×.

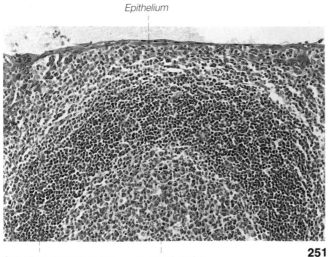

Epithelium

Cap of small lymphocytes   Germinal center

251

Fig. 251. Part of a crypt from a human palatine tonsil. The stratified non-keratinized squamous epithelium is apparently reduced to two or three thin layers since its deeper parts are infiltrated by large numbers of lymphocytes and thereby transformed into a loose cellular, lymphoepithelial network or epithelial reticulum. Below this, parts of a secondary lymphoid nodule with its germinal center and cap of small lymphocytes is visible. H&E staining. Magnification 150×.

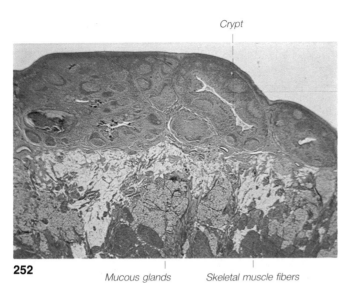

Crypt

252

Mucous glands   Skeletal muscle fibers

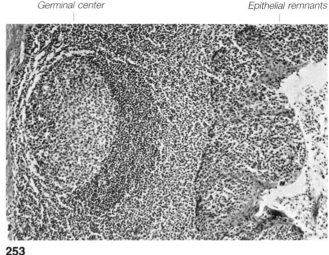

Germinal center   Epithelial remnants

253

Fig. 252. The lingual tonsil, with shorter and less branched crypts than the palatine tonsil, is underlain by numerous predominantly mucous salivary glands and by the skeletal muscle of the tongue. The presence of skeletal muscle near a tonsil is not, however, a specific criterion for its identification (see Fig. 250). Mallory-azan staining. Magnification 12×.

Fig. 253. Close-up of the lower right portion of the crypt indicated in the preceding micrograph by a leader. The crypt epithelium is almost totally transformed into a lymphoepithelial network with only a few recognizable epithelial remnants at its surface. Immediately above the connective tissue there is a secondary lymphoid nodule with a germinal center and crescent cellular cap. Mallory-azan staining. Magnification 96×.

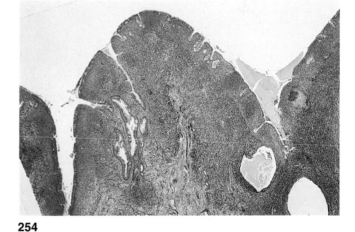

254

Fig. 254. The pharyngeal tonsil is the smallest tonsil and the only one covered by a ciliated pseudostratified columnar epithelium. Well preserved and healthy specimens of this organ are difficult to obtain. It is well-developed only in youth and hence it is only rarely displayed in routine histology courses. Mallory-azan staining. Magnification 14×.

Fig. 255. Higher magnification of the right side of the cone-shaped part of the pharyngeal tonsil shown in the preceding micrograph. The surface respiratory epithelium is easily seen although it is less obvious in the sinuous recesses. Mallory-azan staining. Magnification 96×.

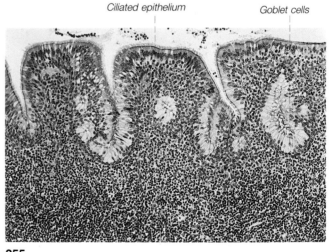

Ciliated epithelium   Goblet cells

255

121

Lymphoid organs – Spleen

Initial identification of the lymphoreticular organs – the lymph nodes, spleen, and thymus – is possible using the naked eye and then a magnifying glass because the lymph nodes and the lobules of the thymus are subdivided into a central medulla and surrounding cortex. In addition only lymph nodes possess a marginal sinus running immediately below the capsule. In contrast the spleen has neither a corticomedullary organization nor a subcapsular sinus, but contains many lymphoid nodules surrounding small arteries known as Malpighian corpuscles. A specific characteristic of the thymus is the presence of medullary bodies (Hassall's corpuscles).

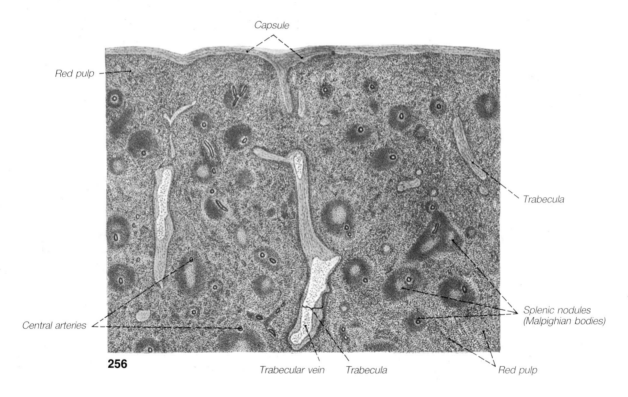

Capsule

Red pulp

Trabecula

Splenic nodules (Malpighian bodies)

Central arteries

256

Trabecular vein *Trabecula* *Red pulp*

Trabecula with trabecular vein

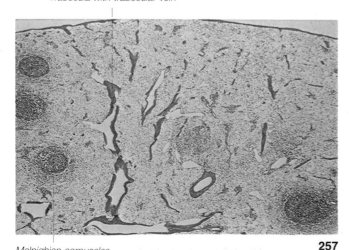

Malpighian corpuscles **257**

Fig. 256. General view of a subcapsular area of human spleen showing several Malpighian corpuscles. These consist of lymphoid tissue with occasional germinal centers forming sleeves around certain divisions of the arteries. They make up the white pulp of the spleen. The arteries in the splenic nodules are called central arteries although they are eccentrically placed within their lymphoid sheaths. The trabeculae, carrying the larger blood vessels and forming a coarse connective tissue framework as they traverse the spleen, are continuous with the fibrous capsule. In some species, e.g., cats, the capsule contains numerous smooth muscle cells (camera lucida drawing). H & E staining. Magnification 22 ×.

Fig. 257. Before fixation the vasculature of this cat spleen was thoroughly lavaged to remove most of the blood it contained. The reticular connective tissue and finer branches of the vascular tree, usually obscured by erythrocytes, are thereby shown more clearly. The Malpighian corpuscles are not affected by this procedure. H & E staining. Magnification 24 ×.

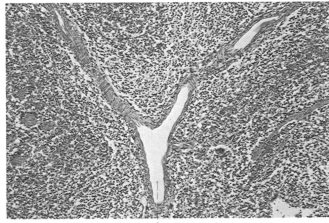

Fig. 258. An artery traversing the splenic red pulp (rhesus monkey). Its two branches extend into the lymphoid tissue sheaths of the white pulp and are thus central arteries of the Malpighian corpuscles. H&E staining. Magnification 95×.

258   *Pulp artery*

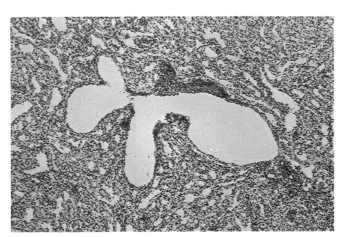

Fig. 259. Low-power micrograph of the red pulp of human spleen showing a trabecular vein with some of its larger tributaries. Mallory-azan staining. Magnification 60×.

259

Lumen of venous sinus   *Reticular fibers*

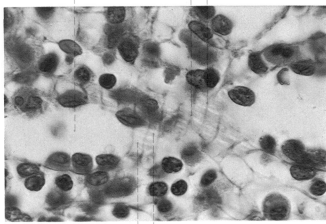

Fig. 260. Only at high magnification is the structural detail of the walls of the venous sinuses seen, particularly when they are cut tangentially (center of this micrograph). The walls consist of elongated, longitudinally arranged endothelial cells (= littoral or lining reticular cells) that stain faintly and are circled by rather coarse reticular fibers. In transverse sections the nuclei of the endothelial cells can be seen bulging into the lumen. Mallory-azan staining. Magnification 960×.

260   *Endothelial cell of venous sinus (long. sec.)*

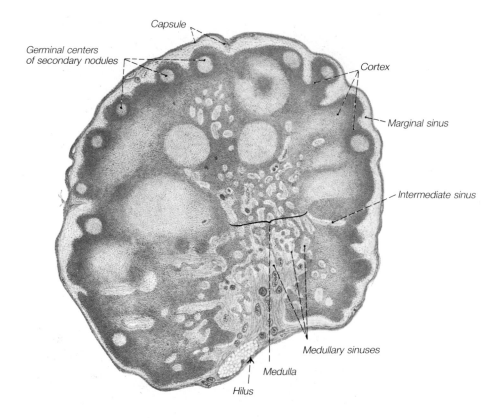

Capsule

Germinal centers
of secondary nodules

Cortex

Marginal sinus

Intermediate sinus

Medullary sinuses

Medulla

Hilus

Fig. 261. Section through an entire human lymph node with an extremely wide subcapsular marginal sinus and an indistinct organization into cortex and medulla. Secondary nodules, i.e., primary nodules in which there is germinal center formation, are mostly restricted to the superficial part of the cortex. The cortex contains many more cells than the medulla and is thus more deeply stained (camera lucida drawing). H & E staining. Magnification 18×.

Medullary sinus

Germinal center

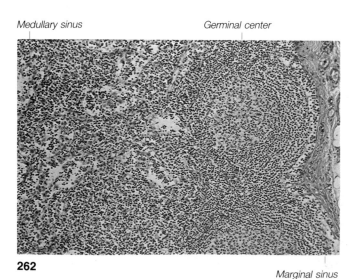

262

Marginal sinus

Fig. 262. Part of a human lymph node at higher magnification. On the right is the fibrous capsule in which several smaller blood vessels can be seen. The underlying narrow marginal sinus is filled with lymphocytes. (The marginal sinus can be very difficult to identify when it is filled with cells as happens in inflammatory reactions and it can also be simulated in the spleen by a subcapsular cleft caused by shrinkage artifact). In the cortex below the marginal sinus is a secondary nodule with its germinal center. The medulla is characterized by numerous, rather broad lymphatic sinuses (= medullary sinuses) with fewer and more loosely arranged cells. Mallory-azan staining. Magnification 95×.

The thymus is characteristically arranged in lobules, each of which is subdivided into cortex and medulla. In addition, the thymus lacks a marginal sinus and secondary nodules, but its medulla contains Hassall's corpuscles.

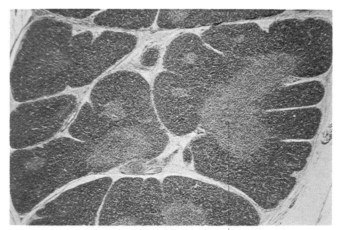

263

Fig. 263. Well-developed thymus of a human fetus showing prominent lobulation and a clear-cut division into cortex and medulla. The cortex is more deeply stained because of its abundance of cells. Hematoxylin-chromotrop staining. Magnification 24×.

Hassal's corpuscle in the medulla

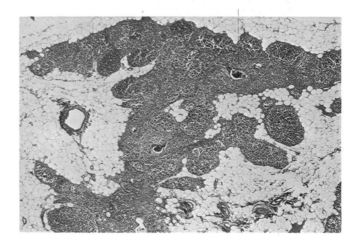

264

Fig. 264. In the thymus of adults the lobulation disappears almost completely due to cortical involution ("age involution"). In the persisting medullary cords, conspicuously large and often cystic Hassall's corpuscles filled with disintegrating material can be found. Hematoxylin-chromotrop staining. Magnification 24×.

Small Hassal's corpuscles　　　*Large Hassal's corpuscle*

Medulla

Fig. 265. Well-developed Hassall's corpuscle from a child's thymus. These bodies are composed of a varying number of concentrically arranged medullary cells and are the most specific characteristic of this lymphoretricular organ. With age they show progressive degeneration of their centers, resulting finally in the formation of cysts (see Fig. 264). Camera lucida drawing. Alum-carmine staining. Magnification 230×.

Cortex

265

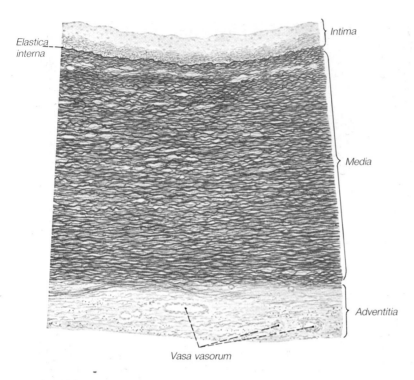

Elastica
interna

Intima

Media

Adventitia

Vasa vasorum

Fig. 266. Segment of a cross-sectioned human aorta with an elastic fiber stain showing the three main tunics which characterize arteries; 1) intima, 2) media, and 3) adventitia composed of connective tissue. When elastic arteries (the aorta with its primary branches and the pulmonary artery) and muscular arteries (see Fig. 273) are compared, it is apparent that the inner and external elastic laminae are less pronounced in the elastic arteries. The smooth muscle cells in the media of this specimen are unstained and hence invisible (camera lucida drawing). Orcein staining. Magnification 60×.

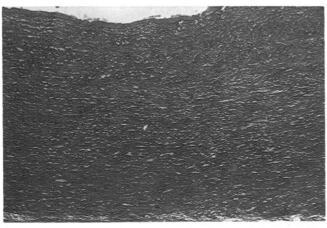

Fig. 267. Low-power view of a cross-sectioned human descending aorta. Histologic sections of aorta are often incorrectly identified as "elastic ligament" or even "smooth muscle tissue" for a variety of reasons; the three tunics are often indistingt in H & E staining, the endothelial layer may have disappeared due to post-mortem changes and the main structural elements of the media (smooth muscle cells and elastic fibers) may be obvious only at higher magnification. H & E staining. Magnification 38×.

267

Vascular lumen

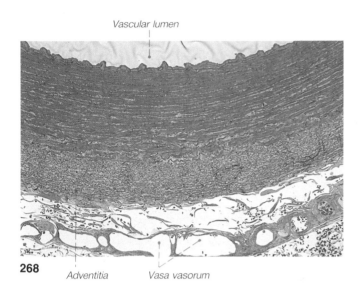

268 Adventitia Vasa vasorum

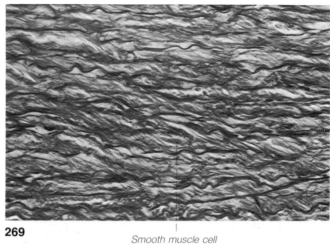

269 Smooth muscle cell

Intimal cells containing lipids Endothelium

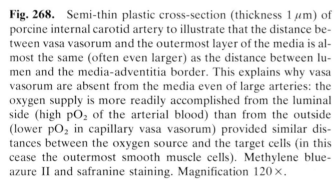

270

Connective tissue beyond the intima Smooth muscle within the intima

Fig. 268. Semi-thin plastic cross-section (thickness 1 μm) of porcine internal carotid artery to illustrate that the distance between vasa vasorum and the outermost layer of the media is almost the same (often even larger) as the distance between lumen and the media-adventitia border. This explains why vasa vasorum are absent from the media even of large arteries: the oxygen supply is more readily accomplished from the luminal side (high pO₂ of the arterial blood) than from the outside (lower pO₂ in capillary vasa vasorum) provided similar distances between the oxygen source and the target cells (in this cease the outermost smooth muscle cells). Methylene blue-azure II and safranine staining. Magnification 120×.

Fig. 269. Aortic media at a higher magnification with a combined stain for cells and elastic fibers to demonstrate the close interrelationships between the muscle cells and the many elastic membranes. The tensile strength of the elastic tissue is regulated by the smooth muscle cells. Staining: Resorcin-fuchsin and azocarmine-naphthol green Magnification 240×.

Fig. 270. Frozen cross-section of porcine external carotid artery from an experimental animal to illustrate early phase of artherosclerosis. The intima is thickened and richer in cells, many of which contain lipids (stained red.). Sudan III and hematoxyline staining. Magnification 150×.

Fig. 271. Segment of the complete thickness of the wall of a cross-sectioned human inferior vena cava. In comparison to the aorta, the components of the caval media are more loosely arranged and separated from the intima by a broad connective tissue layer (subintimal connective tissue). Under its endothelium, the intima contains small strands of smooth muscle cells (staining bright red). Staining: Resorcin-fuchsin and azocarmine-naphthol green. Magnification 95×.

271

Adventitia   Media   Intima   Adipose tissue

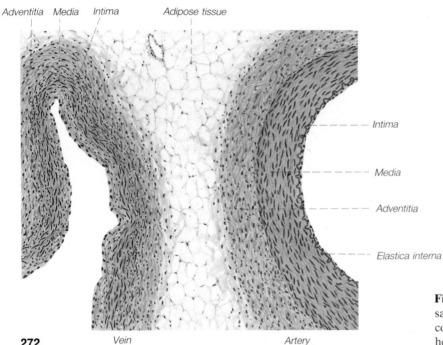

Intima

Media

Adventitia

Elastica interna

272   Vein   Artery

Fig. 272 and 273. Two cross-sections of the same medium-sized muscular artery and its accompanying vein stained, respectively, with hematoxylin-eosin and resorcin-fuchsin to demonstrate the different wall compositions. A reliable criterion for the identification of these vessels is the structure of the media. In arteries this consists of closely apposed smooth muscle cells with only a small number of interspersed connective tissue fibers, whereas the media of veins displays a looser arrangement of fewer muscle cells and a richer supply of collagen fibers. The internal elastic lamina (best seen with elastic stains) is generally more pronounced in arteries than in the corresponding veins, although it may be present in the latter (camera lucida drawing). H & E staining (Fig. 272); resorcin-fuchsin staining (Fig. 273). Magnification 65 ×.

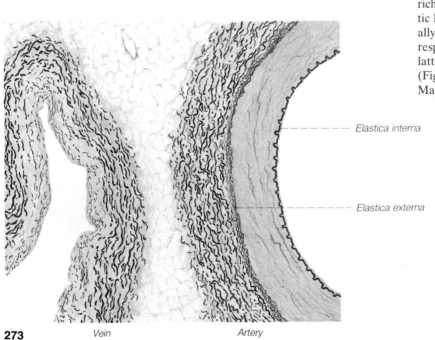

Elastica interna

Elastica externa

273   Vein   Artery

128

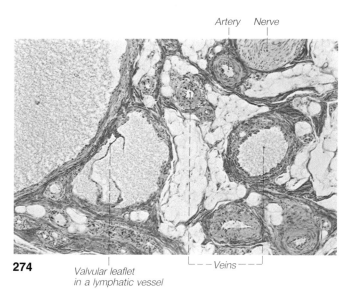

Artery   Nerve

274   *Valvular leaflet in a lymphatic vessel* $\llcorner$ – – *Veins* – – $\lrcorner$

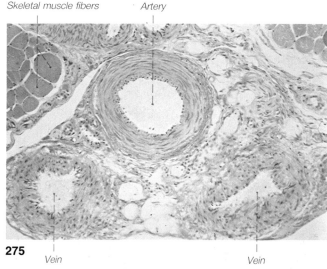

Skeletal muscle fibers   Artery

275   *Vein*   *Vein*

Fig. 274. Low-power view of smaller blood and lymphatic vessels in a human spermatic cord. In this particular location the veins have a media of similar thickness to that of arteries, but the veins can be distinguished by the irregular distribution and smaller number of nuclei within their media (see the following micrograph). The vascular profile filled with proteinaceous material in the upper left corner of the micrograph is a large lymphatic trunk with an adjacent smaller tributary in the lumen of which are the leaflets of a valve. H & E staining. Magnification 60 ×.

Fig. 275. Small muscular artery and its accompanying veins in a human spermatic cord. Although in this particular situation the thickness of the media is similar in arteries and veins, note the difference in both the number and arrangement of the smooth muscle nuclei in the two vessel types. Cross-sectioned skeletal muscle fibers (cremaster muscle) are seen in the upper left corner. H & E staining. Magnification 96 ×.

Fig. 276. Demonstration of capillaries (round "holes") in the rat gastrocnemius muscle by vascular perfusion with a fixative (glutaraldehyde). A classification of muscle fiber types (see Fig. 168) is also possible in this preparation because the semi-thin (0.5 μm) section was subjected to a histochemical method that stains mitochondria and their subsarcolemmal accumulations as brown dots and crescent-shaped areas, respectively. The unusually high capillary number reflects the relatively large number of "red" fibers in this area. *P*-phenylenediamine staining. Magnification 240 ×.

Fig. 277. Larger lymphatic vessel from human subcutaneous tissue together with small arteries and arterioles. When compared to veins of similar size, lymphatics can often be distinguished by the undulating or wavy course of their predominantly endothelial wall. Methylene blue-azure II and safranine staining. Magnification 240 ×.

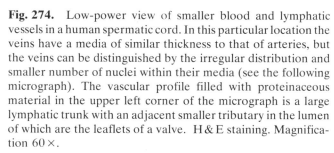

276   *"Red" fiber*   *Blood capillaries*

Mixed peripheral nerve   *Lymphatic vessel*

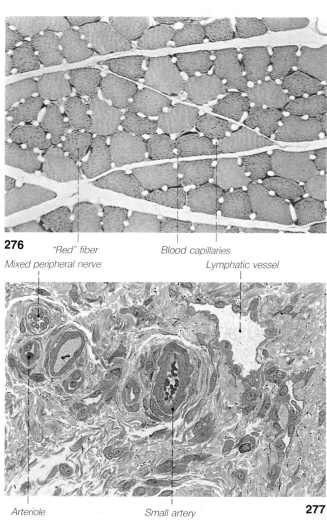

Arteriole   *Small artery*   **277**

129

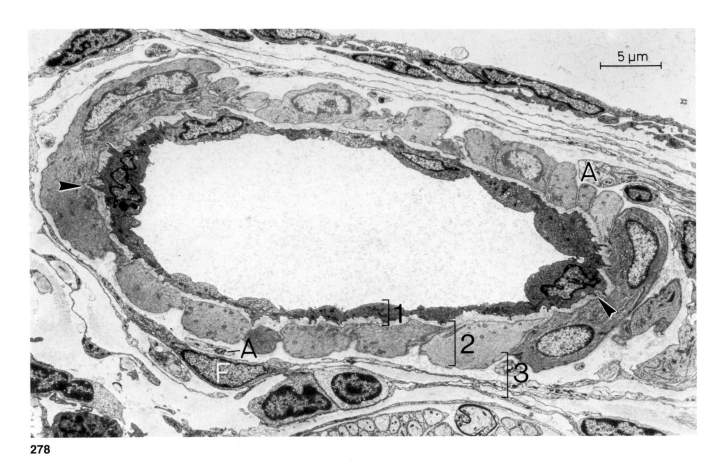

278

Fig. 278.   Slightly oblique section through an arteriole from rat mesentery, showing characteristic three-layered wall texture: (**1**) endothelium with internal elastic lamina (= intima), (**2**) a single layer of smooth muscle cells constituting the media, and (**3**) an outer connective tissue layer, the adventitia. Note basal endothelial projections (►) traversing the internal elastic lamina to establish myoendothelial junctions with the media cells. The adventitia is demarcated from the adjoining loose connective tissue by elongated slender extensions of fibroblasts (**F**) known in this situation as "veil cells". Within the adventitia several bundles of non-myelinated axons (**A**) may be observed. Magnification 3,200×.

Fig. 279.   Transverse section of a capillary of the subcutaneous tissue of a rabbit ear. Because the cytoplasm of the two endothelial cells is uninterrupted, this is an example of a "continuous" capillary. It is almost completely surrounded by the slender process of a pericyte (**3**). Within the endothelial cytoplasm there are groups of vesicles and vacuoles along with a few mitochondria. Mitochondria are also present in the cytoplasm of the pericyte that also contains a well-developed rough ER and numerous free ribosomes. **1** Interendothelial cleft; **2** Basal lamina (►). Magnification 12,500×.

Fig. 280.   Cross-section of a continuous-type capillary from feline myocardium. The flattened portions of the endothelial cells merely display plasmalemmal vesicles (►), the majority of which are continuous with either of the two cell membranes, whereas the thicker parts of the cells also contain several small mitochondria (**1**). Note bundle of non-myelinated axons (**2**), two of which (✳) are partly denuded of Schwann cell cytoplasm where they face and come close to the capillary wall. Arrow indicates interendothelial junction. **3** Cardiomyocyte; **4** T-tubule. Magnification 27,500×.

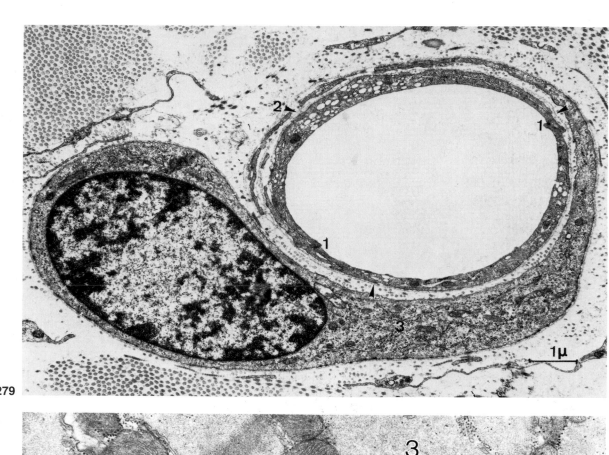

279

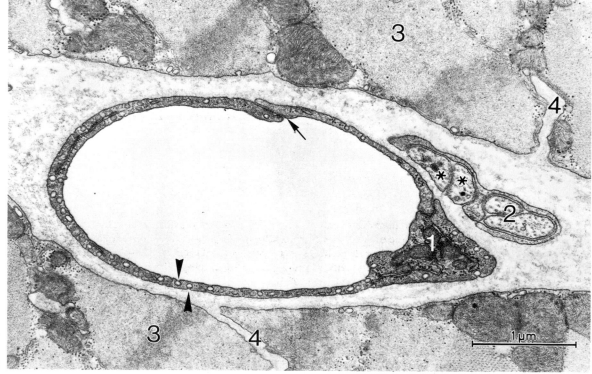

280

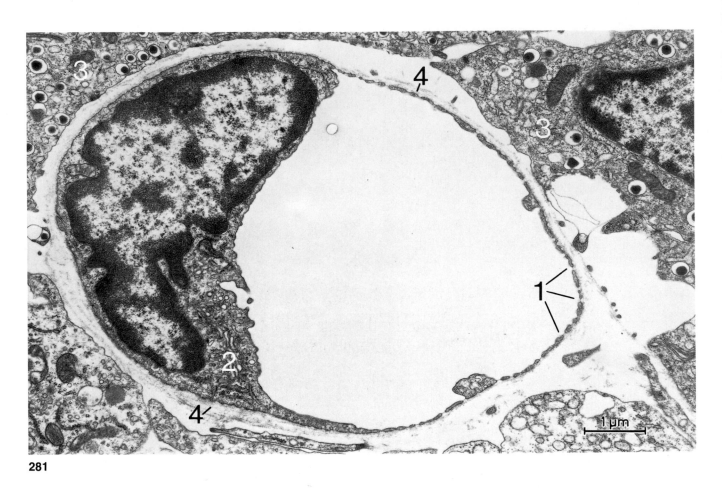

281

Fig. 281. Transverse section of a fenestrated-type capillary from rat pancreatic islet. The endothelium is extremely attenuated over large areas that appear as if perforated by rather regularly spaced openings (**1**). These "fenestrae" are circular pores with a mean diameter ranging between 60 and 80 nm and they are bridged by a delicate membrane, the diaphragm. For detail see Figure 282b. The nucleated portion of the endothelial cytoplasm contains a Golgi complex (**2**). **3** Parts of endocrine cells of the islet; **4** Capillary basal lamina. Magnification 16,000×.

Fig. 282 a). Longitudinal section of a postcapillary venule from feline skeletal muscle (M. soleus) that is continuous with one of its tributaries, the venous segment of a capillary (boxed area in the lower right corner of the venous wall). The latter may be identified by it flattened endothelium fitted with several diaphragmed fenestrae. Magnification 3,500×.
b). Close-up of the boxed area to illustrate attentuated endothelium with fenestrae bridged by a diaphragm. Magnification 38,000×.

Fig. 283. Low-power electron micrograph of a lymphatic vessel from mouse tracheal mucosa. Despite its rather large size this lymphatic displays a capillary wall texture with a characteristically attenuated almost veil-like endothelium. At the junction with a smaller tributary (★) a valve can be seen which consists of two leaflets (**1**) each of which represents a simple endothelial fold projecting into the lumen of the draining vessel. Magnification 2,800×.

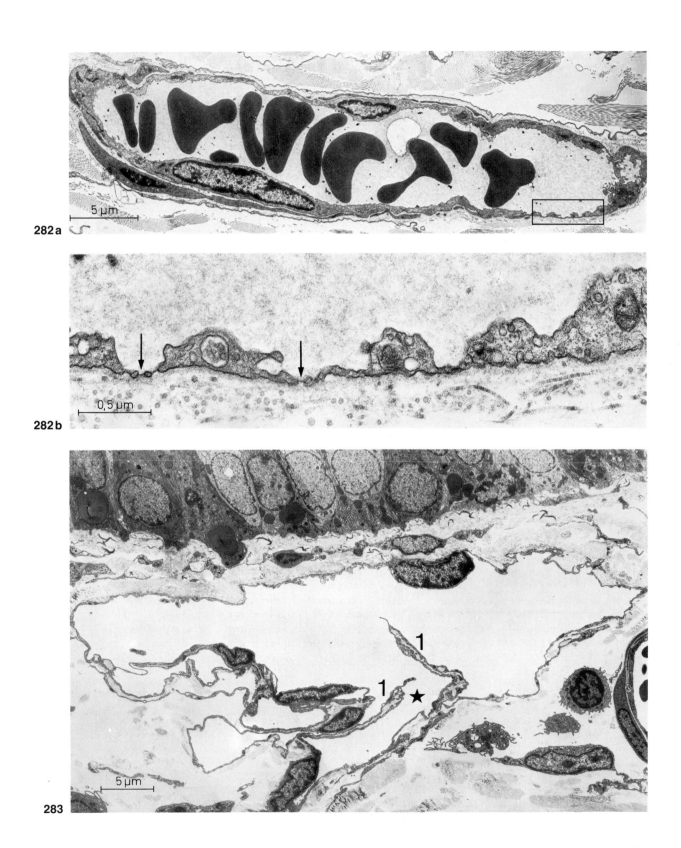

282a

282b

283

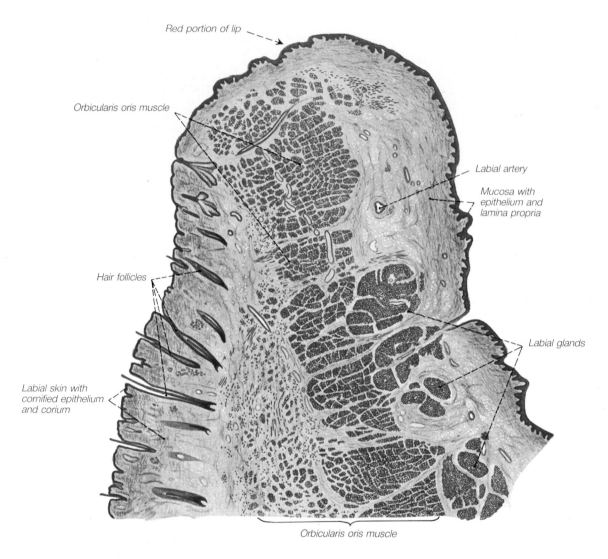

Red portion of lip

Orbicularis oris muscle

Labial artery

Mucosa with epithelium and lamina propria

Hair follicles

Labial glands

Labial skin with cornified epithelium and corium

Orbicularis oris muscle

Fig. 284. The lips are one area of the body characterized, among other features, by a gradual change in the covering epithelium. In this sagittal section it is evident that a typical thin skin with a cornified epithelium, hair follicles and both sweat and sebaceous glands changes in the "red area" (vermilion border) to a noncornified stratified squamous epithelium devoid of glands. This latter epithelium is continuous with the similar noncornified epithelium of the mucous membrane, in the submucosa of which are numerous mixed labial glands. The central core of the lips consists mainly of the striated fibers (cross-sectioned in this specimen) of the orbicularis oris muscle (camera lucida drawing). See Table 11 for comparative identification data. H & E staining. Magnification 8 ×.

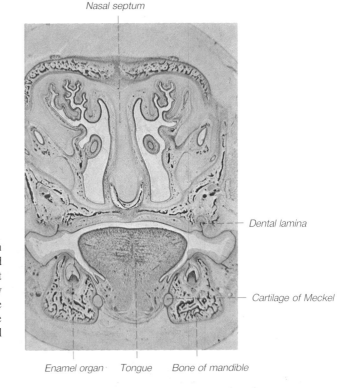

Nasal septum

Dental lamina

Cartilage of Meckel

Enamel organ · Tongue · Bone of mandible

Fig. 285. Frontal section through the snout of a fetal pig. In the upper and lower jaw areas (their osseous trabeculae stained a brilliant blue), tooth germs at different stages of development can be seen. In the maxilla they are represented by the early dental lamina, particularly prominent on the right side of the micrograph. In the mandible they have already reached the stage of the epithelial enamel organs with their mesenchymal dental papillae. Mallory-azan staining. Magnification 9.5 ×.

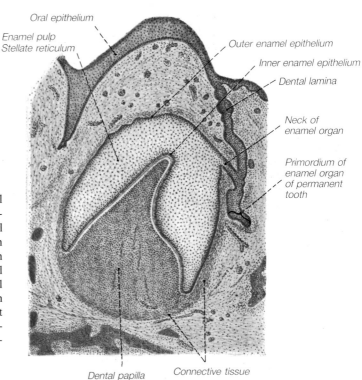

Oral epithelium

Enamel pulp
Stellate reticulum

Outer enamel epithelium

Inner enamel epithelium

Dental lamina

Neck of enamel organ

Primordium of enamel organ of permanent tooth

Fig. 286. At a higher magnification the bell-shaped enamel organ is seen to consist of an inner enamel epithelium (the future enamel-producing ameloblasts) and an outer enamel epithelium adjoining the surrounding mesenchyme. Between the two epithelia is the enamel pulp that consists of a reticulum of epithelial origin that develops from the primary solid enamel organ. The reticulum results from an increase in the interstitial fluid that pushes the epithelial cells apart and transforms them into stellate elements with only their processes still in contact (developing deciduous tooth of a four- to five-month-old human fetus). Camera lucida drawing. H & E staining. Magnification 40 ×.

Dental papilla   Connective tissue

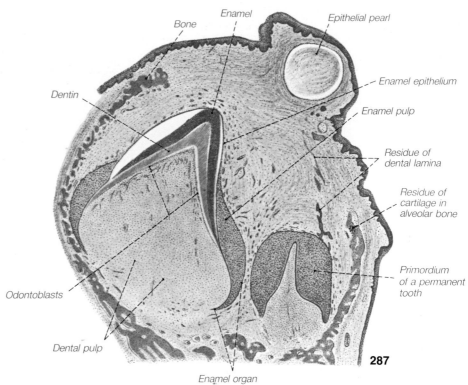

Bone · Enamel · Epithelial pearl

Enamel epithelium

Dentin

Enamel pulp

Residue of dental lamina

Residue of cartilage in alveolar bone

Primordium of a permanent tooth

Odontoblasts

Dental pulp

Enamel organ

287

Fig. 287. Primordia of a deciduous and a permanent tooth of a human neonate, the former already exhibiting deposition of the hard substances, enamel, and dentin. These substances are products of specialized cell types, the amelo- and odontoblasts, and are easily distinguished from each other by their different staining properties (camera lucida drawing). H & E staining. Magnification 12 ×.

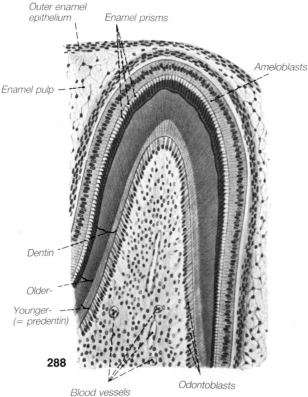

Outer enamel epithelium · Enamel prisms

Ameloblasts

Enamel pulp

Dentin

Older-

Younger-
(= predentin)

288

Blood vessels · Odontoblasts

Fig. 288. Detail from the crown of a human dental primordium (approximate age 6 months) to show the first stages in the deposition of enamel and dentin. The odontoblasts originate from those mesenchymal cells of the dental papilla that are adjacent to the enamel organ. They first produce an uncalcified predentin (= dentinoid) in which cytoplasmic processes (= fibers of Tomes) of the odontoblasts survive and remain active. In contrast the ameloblasts manufacture a secretory product in the form of prisms. As they push the enamel prisms toward the dentin, the cells themselves are moved back from the dentin (camera lucida drawing). H & E staining. Magnification 165 ×.

Fig. 289. Complete longitudinal section through a cat incisor in situ with its crown (the part that projects above the gingiva or gum), neck (the region where enamel and cementum merge) and root (the portion located in the osseous socket or alveolus). In this specimen the enamel is invisible as it was removed during decalcification prior to staining. (camera lucida drawing.) H & E staining. Magnification 10×.

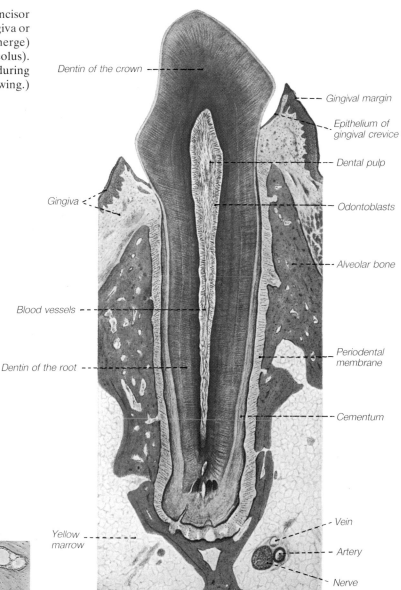

Dentin of the crown

Gingival margin

Epithelium of gingival crevice

Dental pulp

Gingiva

Odontoblasts

Alveolar bone

Blood vessels

Dentin of the root

Periodental membrane

Cementum

Vein

Yellow marrow

Artery

Nerve

289

Connective tissue with blood vessels in the periodental space

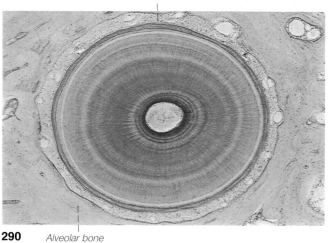

290 Alveolar bone

Fig. 290. Cross-section through a cat incisor in situ. The concentric layering of the dentin is due to its stepwise calcification. The growth lines between the older and more recently formed layers of dentin are known as the contour lines of Owen. Hematoxylin and picric acid staining. Magnification 38×.

Oral cavity – Tongue

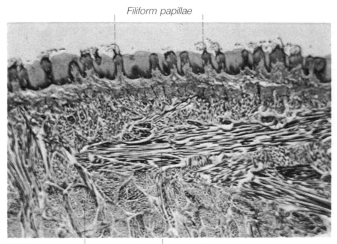

Filiform papillae

291 *Bundles of skeletal muscle fibers*

Fig. 291. Dorsum of human tongue with closely spaced filiform papillae. These consist of a connective tissue core that subdivides into secondary papillae, the covering epithelium of which tapers into thread-like (= filiform) cornifications bent towards the pharynx. These papillae serve a mechanical function. Hematoxylin and azocarmine staining. Magnification 12×.

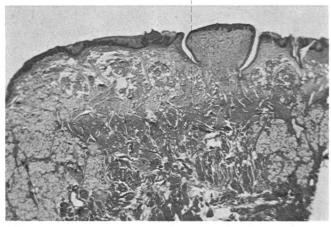

Serous glands

292

Fig. 292. The circumvallate papillae, located at the junction of the dorsum and root of the tongue, are visible with the naked eye. Numerous taste buds are situated in the epithelial walls of their trenches into which open the ducts of the serous glands of von Ebner. At this low magnification the taste buds cannot be identified. H & E staining. Magnification 12×.

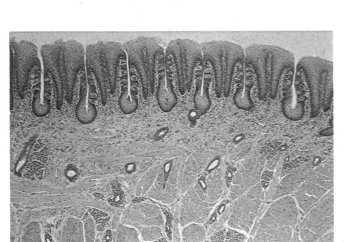

293

Fig. 293. The foliate papillae are only poorly developed in man, but well developed in a number of animal species such as the rabbit. At the posterolateral aspect of the tongue they form an oval area, the foliate region, consisting of slender mucosal folds oriented perpendicularly to the lingual border. The epithelium lining the trenches of these papillae is particularly rich in taste buds that at low magnifications appear as cone-shaped translucencies due to their poor stainability (for details cf. Figs. 498 and 499). Iron hematoxylin staining. Magnification 38×.

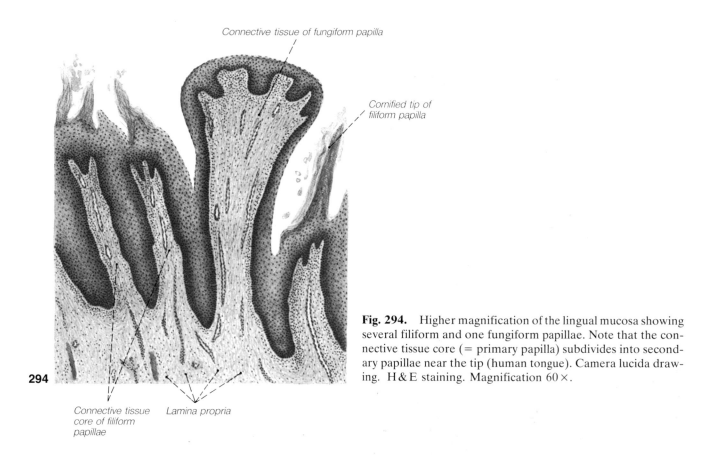

Connective tissue of fungiform papilla

Cornified tip of
filiform papilla

294

Connective tissue
core of filiform
papillae

Lamina propria

Fig. 294. Higher magnification of the lingual mucosa showing
several filiform and one fungiform papillae. Note that the connective tissue core (= primary papilla) subdivides into secondary papillae near the tip (human tongue). Camera lucida drawing. H & E staining. Magnification 60 ×.

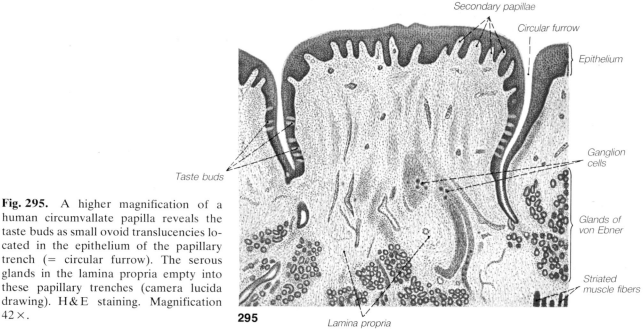

Secondary papillae

Circular furrow

Epithelium

Ganglion
cells

Glands of
von Ebner

Striated
muscle fibers

Taste buds

Fig. 295. A higher magnification of a
human circumvallate papilla reveals the
taste buds as small ovoid translucencies located in the epithelium of the papillary
trench (= circular furrow). The serous
glands in the lamina propria empty into
these papillary trenches (camera lucida
drawing). H & E staining. Magnification
42 ×.

295

Lamina propria

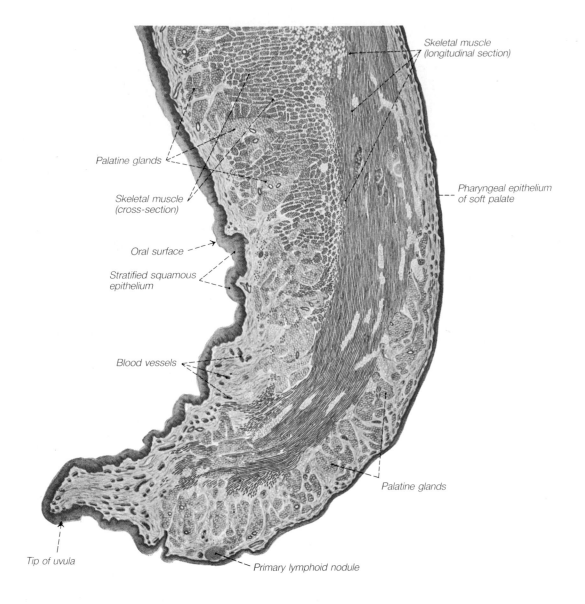

Skeletal muscle
(longitudinal section)

Palatine glands

Skeletal muscle
(cross-section)

Pharyngeal epithelium
of soft palate

Oral surface

Stratified squamous
epithelium

Blood vessels

Palatine glands

Tip of uvula

Primary lymphoid nodule

Fig. 296. Longitudinal section through the soft palate and uvula. As in the lips, the central tissue core at this site consists mainly of striated muscle fibers. Unlike the lips, however, the covering of both the palatine and pharyngeal surfaces is a noncornified stratified squamous epithelium which changes only in its height. Its point of continuity with the respiratory epithelium of the nasal cavity is not, as is widely assumed, at the free margin, but on the pharyngeal surface and often (as in this specimen) so far up as not to be included in the section (camera lucida drawing). See Table 11 for comparative identification data. H & E staining. Magnification 7.5×.

The three large salivary glands of the oral cavity, the parotid, the submandibular and the sublingual glands, differ in both the type of their secretory units and the organization and composition of their duct systems. The duct systems are particularly useful in discriminating these glands from other similar exocrine glands, such as the lacrimal gland or the pancreas (see Figs. 307–309 and Table 12).

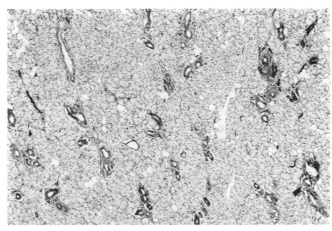

297

Fig. 297. Low-power view of the exclusively serous human parotid gland in which the large number of duct profiles – in this specimen predominantly striated (salivary) ducts – is particularly striking and best evaluated with the lowest power objective of the microscope. The large number of duct profiles is an essential criterion for distinguishing the parotid gland from both the pancreas and the lacrimal gland. In the connective tissue between the secretory alveoli, fat cells are often seen, as they may be in other salivary glands. Characteristic of the parotid gland, though not found in every specimen, are profiles of larger nerve bundles that are ramifications of the facial nerve. Mallory-azan staining. Magnification 42 ×.

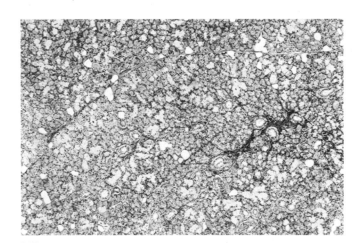

298

Fig. 298. Even at a low magnification the mixed human submandibular gland clearly exhibits both the different stainability of its secretory units and the less well-developed duct system when compared with the parotid gland. With the Mallory-azan stain the mucous tubules present a light bluish appearance, while with H & E they remain more or less unstained and hence appear "white". Mallory-azan staining. Magnification 42 ×.

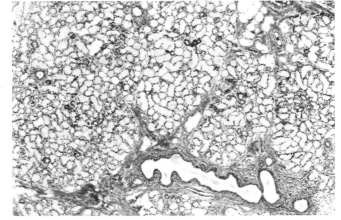

299

Fig. 299. The human sublingual gland is also a mixed gland, although it is predominantly mucous. Because of the large number and poor stainability of the mucous tubules, the beginner may consider them to be serous units thereby missing the mixed nature of the gland. The sublingual gland has even fewer duct profiles than the submandibular gland. Mallory-azan staining. Magnification 42 ×.

Salivary (striated) duct   Intercalated duct

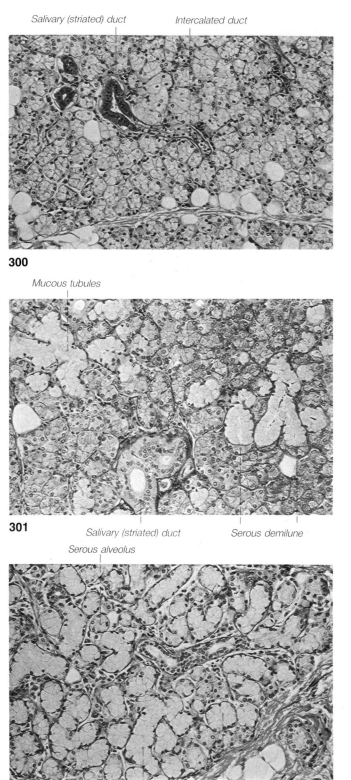

Capillary   Small artery

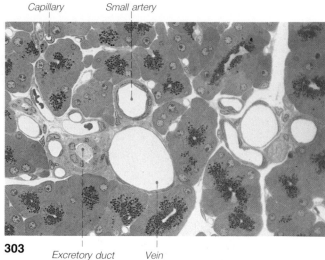

300

Mucous tubules

301

Salivary (striated) duct   Serous demilune

Serous alveolus

302   Mucous tubules

303   Excretory duct   Vein

Fig. 300. The secretory units of the human parotid gland can be identified only at higher magnifications. They are of different sizes because they consist of a varying number of secretory cells. Their nuclei always show a rounded outline and are usually found at the cell base due to the massive accumulation of secretory products (see also Figs. 103, 111 and 304). In the center of the micrograph a longitudinally sectioned intercalated duct continues into a cross-sectioned and deeper staining striated (salivary) duct. Mallory-azan staining. Magnification 150×.

Fig. 301. In the submandibular gland the mucous tubules stand out from the usually berry-shaped serous secretory units (acini) by their different stainability, their flattened basally situated nuclei and their tubular shape. In many places the blind ends of the mucous tubules are capped by crescent groups of serous cells, the demilunes of von Ebner or crescents of Giannuzzi. Mallory-azan staining. Magnification 150×.

Fig. 302. The large number of mucous tubules found in the human sublingual gland at first sight seem to indicate homogeneity of the secretory units, but both distinct serous demilunes and "free" serous units (i.e., not associated with the mucous tubules) show that this is not the case. Mallory-azan staining. Magnification 150×.

Fig. 303. Semi-thin plastic section (thickness 1μm) to demonstrate cytological details of secretory units, duct system, and blood vessels. The apical portions of the secretory cells are crowded with zymogen granules, the basal portions are closely approximated to capillaries appearing as empty holes. A larger vein, its corresponding artery on top is accompanied by an excretory duct. Methylene blue-azure II and safranine staining. Magnification 240×.

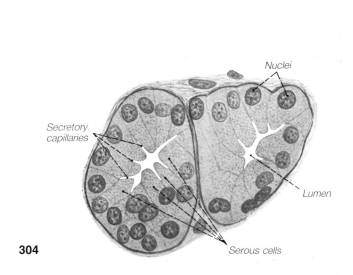

304

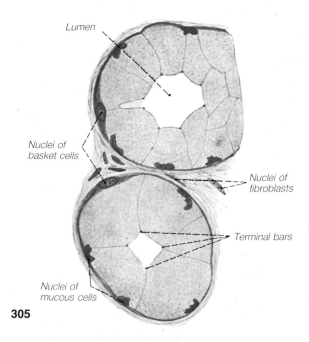

305

Figs. 304–306. Camera lucida drawings showing the cellular details of different secretory units from human salivary glands at the same magnification (oil immersion, 750×) and with same stain (H & E). Whereas at lower magnifications (see Fig. 300) the serous secretory units seem to lack lumina, here (Fig. 304) the narrow slit-like lumina are visualized. The nuclei of the serous cells are always circular in outline and situated towards the base of the cell. The lumina of the mucous tubules (Fig. 305) are usually much larger, although they may be difficult to detect because the secretion they contain often obscures the apical surfaces of the cells. The nuclei of these mucous-producing cells are always flattened against the cell base and have an irregular outline. In the mixed glands (Fig. 306) the serous cells usually line the blind ends of the mucous tubules in the shape of a crescent, the serous demilunes of von Ebner. The aqueous secretion of the serous cells dilutes the mucus, thus lowering its viscosity and enhancing its flow velocity. Intercellular canaliculi or secretory capillaries course between adjacent serous cells.

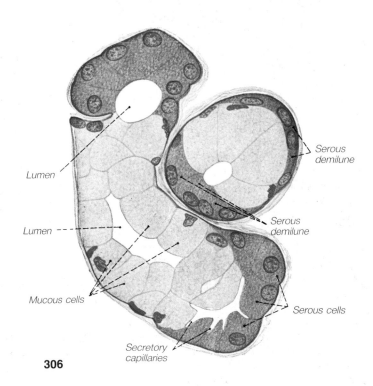

306

Serous glands – Differential diagnosis

Different segments of the duct system

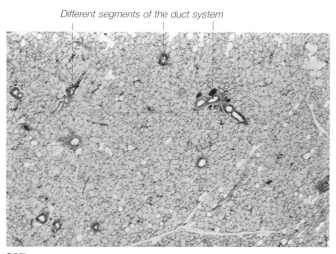

307

Excretory duct   *Islet*

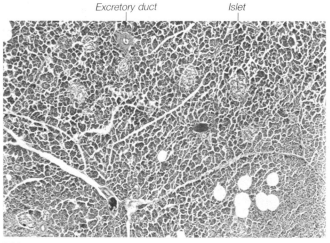

308

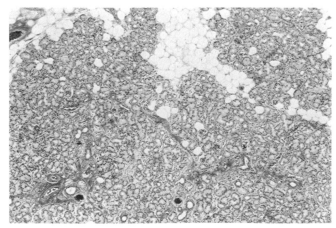

309

Figs. 307–309. The precise identification of the large serous glands – the parotid gland (Fig. 307), the pancreas (Fig. 308), and the lacrimal gland (Fig. 309) – is best achieved by the use of a low-power objective and not, as is often believed, by means of structural details such as the centro-acinar cells of the pancreas.

The best and near crucial criterion for identifying the parotid gland is the larger number of duct profiles always present, which readily distinguish this gland from the other two.

The identification of the pancreas is based on:
1) the islets of Langerhans, also best seen at low magnification because of their lighter staining than the exocrine components.
2) The occurrence of only a few excretory ducts that are always interlobular in position.
3) The poorly developed interlobular connective tissue septa. Even when islets are not present in a section (the head and uncinate process are almost devoid of islets), the first two criteria are enough for the unequivocal identification of the pancreas.

The lacrimal gland is easily distinguished by the rather large and thus prominent lumina of its secretory units, which are also more loosely arranged than those in the pancreas and parotid gland.
All Figures: Mallory-azan staining. Magnification 42×.

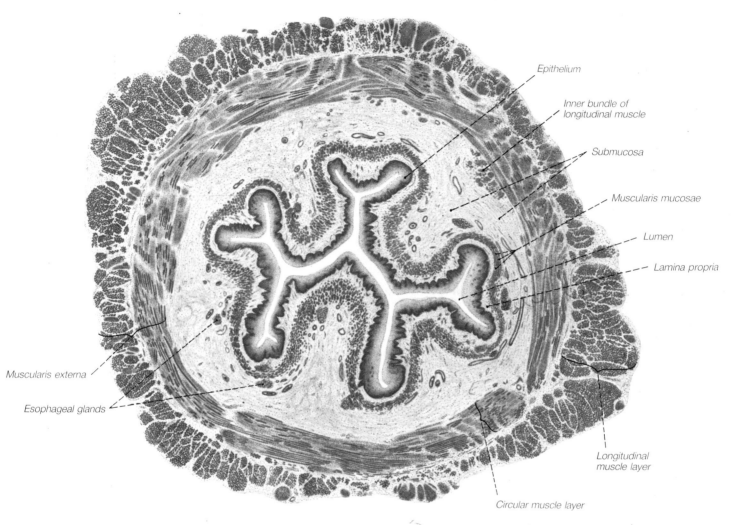

Epithelium

Inner bundle of longitudinal muscle

Submucosa

Muscularis mucosae

Lumen

Lamina propria

Muscularis externa

Esophageal glands

Longitudinal muscle layer

Circular muscle layer

Fig. 310. Camera lucida drawing of a complete cross-section of a human esophagus. The characteristic structure of the wall is shared in basically similar fashion by the remainder of the alimentary tract.
The wall consists of:
1) A mucosa composed of an epithelial lining with a lamina propria made of loose, often reticular connective tissue and a muscularis mucosae. This is a smooth muscle layer of varying thickness that is the most distinctive feature of the entire alimentary tract.
2) A connective tissue submucosa and, finally,
3) A muscularis externa. The muscularis externa is always subdivided into an inner circular and an outer longitudinal layer, with the autonomic myenteric plexus lying in between.
The disposition of these two muscle layers in any section allows one to decide whether the specimen has been cut in cross- or longitudinal section, e.g., in a cross-section the inner circular layer will be cut longitudinally.
The presence of a muscularis mucosae not only clearly demonstrates that the esophagus belongs to the alimentary tract, but also distinguishes this organ from other regions which show the same type of stratified noncornified squamous epithelium, such as the oral cavity, the cornea, the external urethral orifice, the vagina, and the uterine ectocervix. In case of doubt, the presence of small glands within its submucosa will differentiate the esophagus from such structures as the vagina, but since these glands are widely spaced and few in number, their absence does not rule against the identification of "esophagus" if all the other criteria are satisfied. The esophagus differs from other parts of the alimentary tract, all of which possess a simple columnar epithelium. H & E staining. Magnification 11×.

Gastric pits   Muscularis mucosae

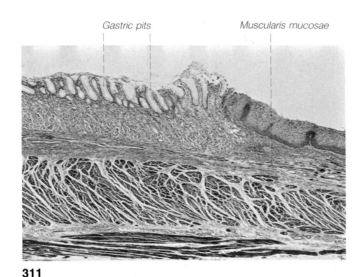

311

Fig. 311. Longitudinal section (because the outer muscular layer is cut longitudinally) through the human cardia, the esophagogastric junction. Note the characteristic abrupt change from a stratified noncornified squamous epithelium to a simple columnar one and the occurrence of epithelial crypts (= gastric pits) that are continuous with the tubular gastric glands found in the deeper mucosal layers. Mallory-azan staining. Magnification 19×.

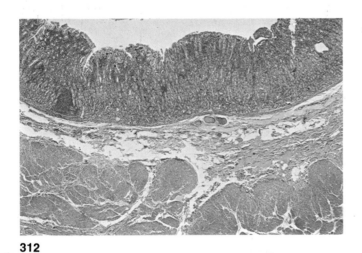

312

Fig. 312. Longitudinal section of human gastric fundus. The closely spaced secretory tubules of the mucosa empty into gastric pits that here are relatively shallow in comparison to the total mucosal height. The thin muscularis mucosae is indistinguishable at this low magnification. A reliable distinction between the gastric fundus and the colon, with which it is often confused, is the fact that goblet cells are never found in the stomach, but always occur in large numbers in the colonic crypts (cf. Figs. 102, 326). H & E staining. Magnification 19×.

Gastric pits   Lymphoid nodule

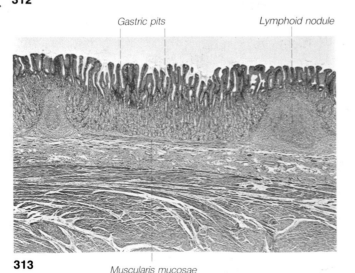

313

Muscularis mucosae

Fig. 313. Compared to the gastric fundus, the epithelial pits of the pyloric mucosa are much deeper, thus occupying a greater proportion of the total mucosal thickness. They are therefore more readily recognized. As in many other mucosae, lymphoid aggregates of various sizes are found amongst the secretory tubules of the pyloric glands. They should not be confused with the focal aggregates of lymphoid nodules found in the submucosa of the ileum. In this specimen, the larger of the lymphoid aggregates (on the right side of the micrograph) has a germinal center and is thus a lymphoid follicle. Hematoxylin and chromotrop staining. Magnification 19×.

Besides possessing the four wall layers characteristic of the entire alimentary tract, the three successive parts of the small intestine (duodenum, jejunum, and ileum) show a particular arrangement of their mucosal surfaces, namely the simultaneous occurrence of folds and villi. The folds (= valves of Kerckring or plicae circulares) are easily seen with the naked eye and comprise not only the entire mucosa, but also parts of the submucosa, the latter constituting a central connective tissue core.

The villi are much smaller finger-like projections of the mucosa only, seen with the aid of a magnifying glass or low power objective. Since the folds decrease in number toward the ileum, specimens of this part of the small intestine may not contain folds (see Fig. 316). The absence of folds does not preclude an identification of "ileum" if all other criteria support it. To include as many of the circularly oriented folds as possible in a section, specimens of small intestine are normally cut longitudinally. Folds may be absent in transverse sections, emphasizing how important it is always to decide first in which planes the two layers of the muscularis externa are cut (for differentiation, see Table 13).

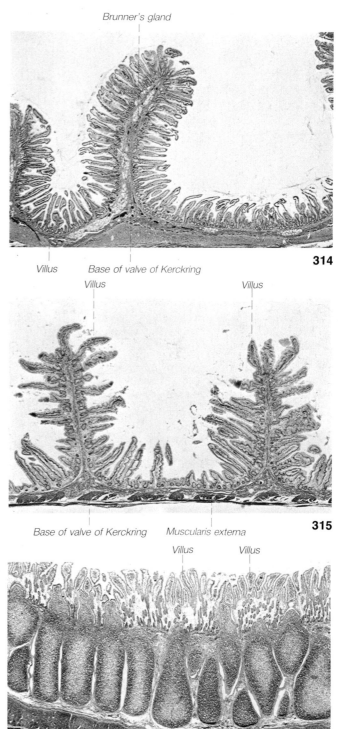

Fig. 314. Longitudinal section of the human duodenum. Note how the entire mucosal surface, including that of the folds, is covered with closely spaced villi. The palely stained areas of the submucosa are the glands of Brunner, unique to the duodenum and clearly differentiating it from the other segments of the small intestine. Mallory-azan staining. Magnification 12×.

Fig. 315. Longitudinal section through a human jejunum with two of its folds. The submucosa is devoid of glands. Due to a varying degree of shrinkage artifact, several villi show translucent clefts between their epithelium and connective tissue core. Mallory-azan staining. Magnification 21.5×.

Fig. 316. Though cut longitudinally, none of the widely spaced folds has been included in this specimen of human ileum. The villi only occasionally contain large artifactual clefts. The most characteristic identifying feature of the ileum is the aggregation of lymphoid nodules (= Peyer's patches) in the submucosa. Mallory-azan staining. Magnification 14.5×.

147

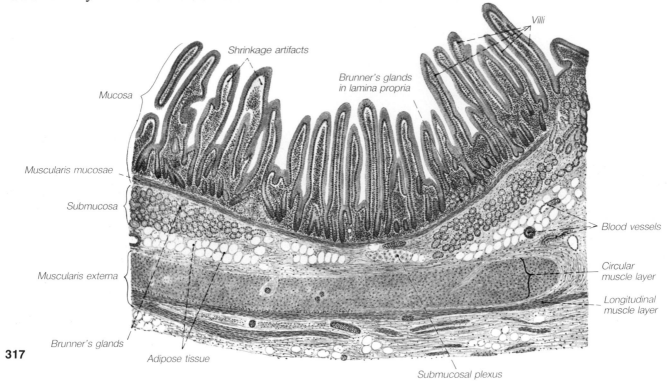

317

Fig. 317. A higher magnification of the human duodenal mucosa shows that the simple columnar epithelium not only covers the villi, but also lines tubular invaginations (= crypts of Lieberkühn), the blind ends of which reach the muscularis mucosae. These crypts are found not only in the duodenum, but also in the other parts of the small intestine, the entire length of which is thus characterized by folds, villi, and crypts. H & E staining. Magnification 50 ×.

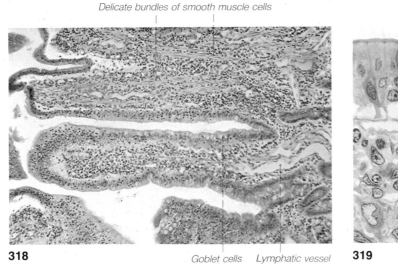

318

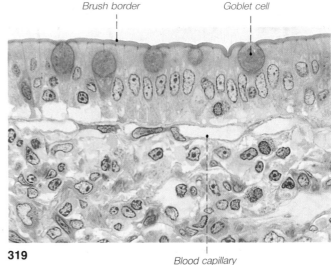

319

Fig. 318. Higher magnification of the jejunal villi of a cat show goblet cells as lighter-staining ellipsoids scattered throughout the epithelium. The delicate smooth muscle bundles stretching from the muscularis mucosae into the connective tissue cores of the villi are responsible for the retraction of the villi during their motile activity, the "villous pump". The intestinal lumen is at the left side of the micrograph. H & E staining. Magnification 96 ×.

Fig. 319. Since biopsies taken for diagnostic purposes from different parts of the digestive canal are also studied with the electron microscope, a semi-thin section (thickness approx. 0.5 μm) as is routinely prepared in electron microscopic laboratories is shown in this micrograph (from guinea pig jejunum). The striated (brush) border appears as a dark blue line with the stain applied. The goblet cells also stand out clearly as deeply colored roundish corpuscles. Note capillaries closely attached to the epithelial basal lamina and the highly cellular reticular connective tissue representing the lamina propria. Methylene blue-azure II staining. Magnification 600 ×.

Parietal cell

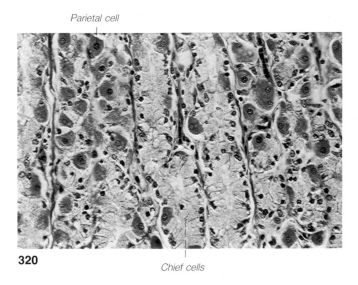

320

Chief cells

Smooth muscle cells in lamina propria of a villus

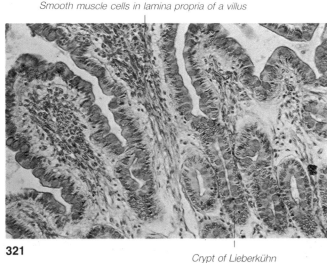

321

Crypt of Lieberkühn

Fig. 320. Unlike the pyloric glands, the secretory tubules of the human gastric fundus are equipped with acidophilic parietal cells, colored brownish-red in this specimen. Attached to the outer surface of the glandular tubules, these cells secrete the ionized hydrogen necessary for the production of hydrochloric acid. Since parietal cells may be difficult to visualize because of faded or nonspecific, e.g., H&E staining, the identification of the gastric fundus should be based on the structure of the whole mucosa (see Fig. 312). Iron hematoxylin and thiazine red staining. Magnification 240×.

Fig. 321. Villi and crypts of the human ileum, the epithelium of which contains numerous goblet cells (stained blue). Within the villous stroma, note the slender elongated smooth muscle cells that form loose aggregates that splay out like a fountain as they approach the tip of the villus. Mallory-azan staining. Magnification 150×.

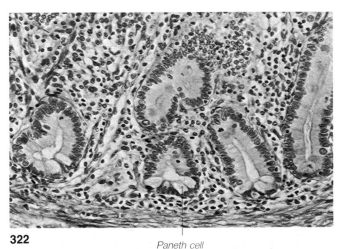

322

Paneth cell

Reticular connective tissue of lamina propria

Fig. 322. Obliquely, transversely, and longitudinally sectioned crypts within the lamina propria of the human duodenal mucosa. In the depths of the crypts are the secretory cells of Paneth which produce, among others, the proteinaceous bacteriolytic enzyme, lysozyme. Mallory-azan staining. Magnification 240×.

Fig. 323. Cross-section through the crypts of the colonic mucosa. Unlike that of the small intestine, the mucosa of the large intestine has no villi although it does show these regularly spaced invaginations (see Fig. 102). Note that in contrast to villi, where the epithelium encircles a connective tissue core, the crypt epithelium surrounds a central opening or lumen. The goblet cells appear as ovoid translucencies within the epithelial lining. H&E staining. Magnification 150×.

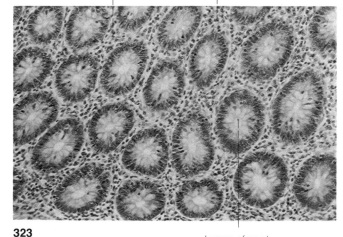

323

Lumen of crypt

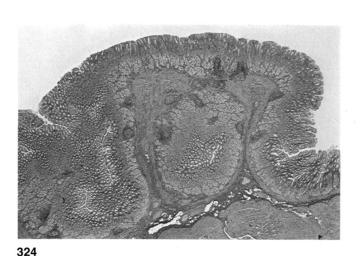

324

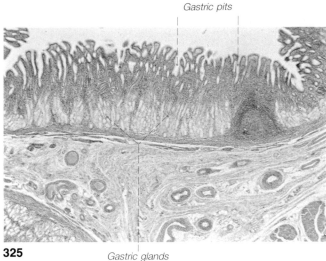

Gastric pits

325

Gastric glands

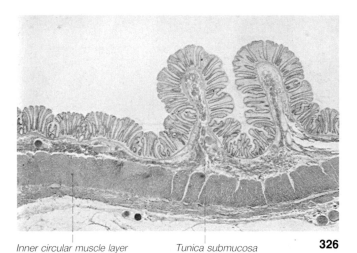

Inner circular muscle layer   *Tunica submucosa*   **326**

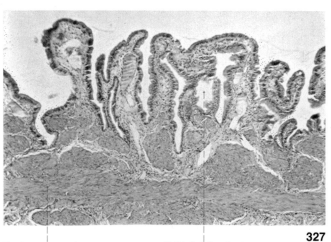

Tunica muscularis   *Epithelial diverticulum of crypt*   **327**

Figs. 324–327. A comparison of various parts of the alimentary tract that are often confused with each other or misinterpreted. Although the stomach may show folds (Fig. 324), these are much coarser than those of the small intestine. The pyloric portion (Fig. 325) is distinguished from the fundus (Fig. 324) by 1) its deeper gastric pits, occupying about half the mucosal thickness, and 2) its more loosely packed tubular glands. The whole stomach can be distinguished from the colon (Fig. 326), with which it is often confused, by the overall greater thickness of its wall, particularly notable in the muscularis externa and by the occurrence of goblet cells in the colonic mucosa.

Although the large intestine (Fig. 326) may also have folds, its mucosa lacks the villi characteristic of the small intestine and the elongated branched tubular glands of the stomach, consisting instead of regularly arranged crypts in whose epithelium numerous goblet cells are interspersed (see also Fig. 102).

The gallbladder (Fig. 327) often remains unrecognized because it is not considered when one is dealing with the identification of the various parts of the alimentary tract to which it belongs only in a wider sense. The gallbladder is characterized by 1) the absence of a muscularis mucosae, 2) a muscularis that is not subdivided into two distinct layers, and 3) many irregular narrow mucosal folds. The folds interconnect with one another, producing irregular polygonal depressions in between, so that a section of gallbladder gives the impression of epithelial cavities (= diverticula) of various sizes enclosed within anastomosing folds.

H & E staining (Figs. 324, 325 and 327). Mallory-azan staining (Fig. 326). Magnifications 9, 11, 13.5 and 48 ×, respectively.

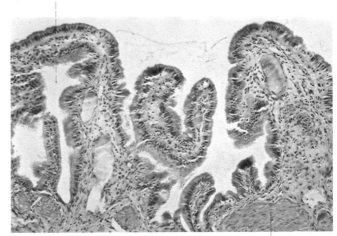

Epithelial diverticulum in a mucosal fold

Fig. 328. At a higher magnification, it can be seen that the simple columnar epithelium of the human gallbladder consists of particularly tall cells and is completely devoid of goblet cells. The muscularis, composed of interlacing bundles of smooth muscle, is separated from the epithelial lining by a poorly defined lamina propria. H & E staining. Magnification 96 ×.

328

Innermost layer of muscular tunic

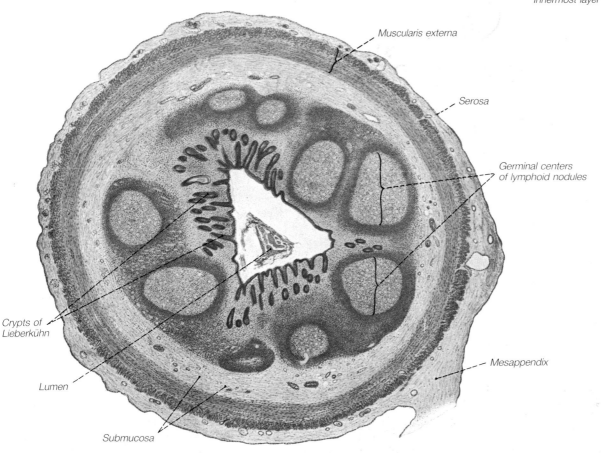

Muscularis externa

Serosa

Germinal centers of lymphoid nodules

Crypts of Lieberkühn

Mesappendix

Lumen

Submucosa

Fig. 329. Complete transverse section through the human vermiform appendix. The mucosa closely resembles that of the colon although its crypts are not as regularly spaced and may be partly missing. Particularly striking are the numerous lymphoid nodules scattered through the lamina propria and reaching into the submucosa. The lymphoid nodules displace the crypts to varying extents and infiltrate and disrupt the thin muscularis mucosae, making this layer difficult to discern (camera lucida drawing). H & E staining. Magnification 22 ×.

151

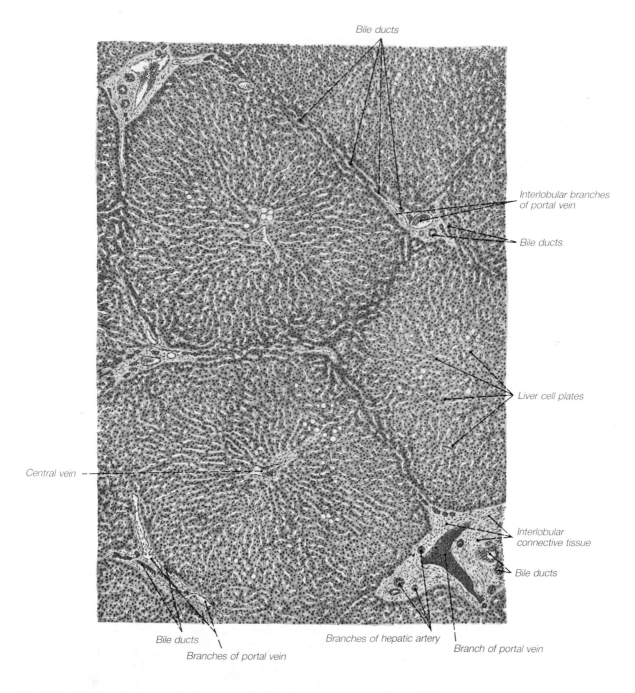

Bile ducts

Interlobular branches
of portal vein

Bile ducts

Liver cell plates

Central vein

Interlobular
connective tissue

Bile ducts

Bile ducts

Branches of hepatic artery

Branch of portal vein

Branches of portal vein

Fig. 330. The liver is composed of innumerable hepatic lobules, the outlines of which have been specially emphasized in this camera lucida drawing in order to demonstrate the organization of these structural units more clearly than is usually seen in man. In sections these lobules appear as rounded or polygonal units consisting of 1) hepatic cells arranged in plates or cords radiating around a central blood vessel (= central vein) and 2) interconnecting liver sinusoids which lie between the hepatic plates. Connective tissue between the lobules is only clearly apparent where three or more lobules meet, a point known as a portal canal or area. These canals regularly contain the interlobular bile duct along with branches of the portal vein and hepatic artery, the duct and two vessel types forming the "portal triad". H & E staining. Magnification 70 ×.

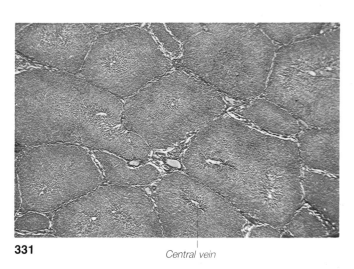

331   *Central vein*

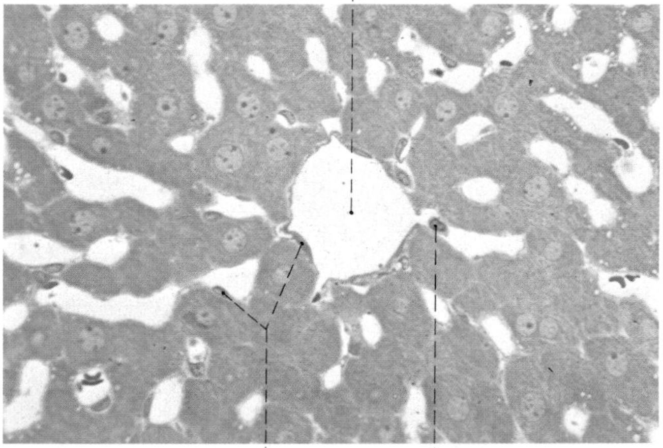

Central vein

332   *Endothelial nuclei*   *Nucleus of a Kupffer cell*

Fig. 331. In the pig liver the hepatic lobules are particularly well demarcated because each is completely surrounded by connective tissue septa. Specimens from this species are thus often chosen to introduce the student to the lobular organization of the liver. Mallory-azan staining. Magnification 19 ×.

333

Fig. 332. The center of a rat hepatic lobule shown in a semithin section. Because such sections are only 0.5–1 μm thick and the tissue better fixed (in this experimental animal by vascular perfusion), specimens like this reveal much more structural detail than those obtained by conventional methods. Note the distinct endothelial nuclei in the sinusoids and central vein. Methylene blue-azure II staining. Magnification 380 ×.

Fig. 333. Detail of a human hepatic lobule showing the delicate network of reticular fibers enmeshing the liver cells and emphasizing their radial arrangement around the central vein. Silver impregnation. Magnification 95 ×.

Hepatic artery

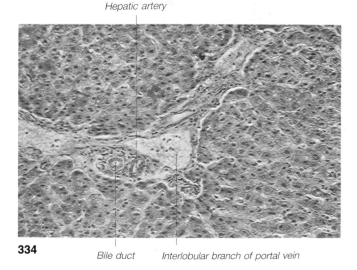

Fig. 334. Portal canal from a human liver. The individual components of the "portal triad" – interlobular bile duct and branches of the portal vein and hepatic artery – are easily distinguished by their differing wall structure. H & E staining. Magnification 150 ×.

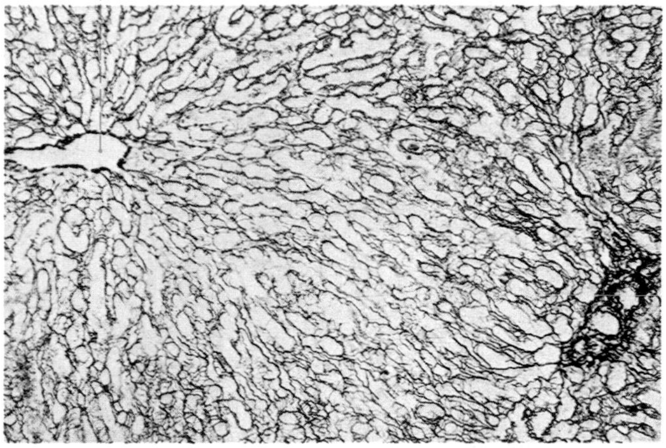

334   *Bile duct*   *Interlobular branch of portal vein*

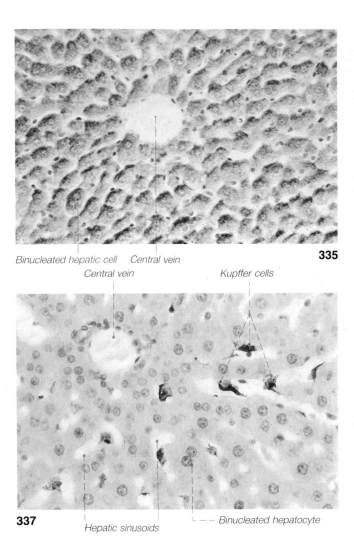

Binucleated hepatic cell   Central vein   **335**
Central vein   Kupffer cells

Vacuoles within hepatic cells   Kupffer cell nucleus

336   Hepatic nucleolus

337
Hepatic sinusoids   └ – – Binucleated hepatocyte

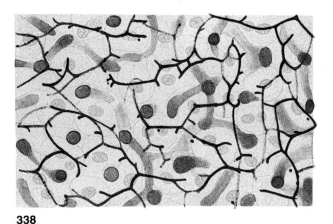

338

Fig. 335. Hepatic cell cords showing intracellular glycogen deposits in the form of granules of various sizes (see also Fig. 53). PAS and hemalum staining. Magnification 240×.

Fig. 336. Semi-thin section of liver parenchyma with several sinusoids. The hepatocytes show several, possibly artifactual vacuoles along those surfaces adjoining the space of Disse. Note the delicate endothelium and the nucleus of a Kupffer cell in the longitudinally sectioned sinusoid on the right (cf. Figs. 340 and 341). Methylene blue-azure II staining. Magnification 960×.

Fig. 337. The stellate-shaped cells of Kupffer, located within the liver sinusoids, belong to the reticuloendothelial (mononuclear phagocytic) system. They can only be seen with the light microscope after their intense phagocytic capacity has been employed to "mark" the cells with ingested foreign material, e.g., intravitally injected with trypan blue or colloidal silver. Note binucleated hepatocytes. Technique: colloidal silver intravitally, counterstained with nuclear fast red. Magnification 380×.

Fig. 338. The three-dimensional networks formed by the bile "capillaries" and the hepatic sinusoids demonstrated by injection of differently colored gelatin solutions (camera lucida drawing). The blackish colored minute bile canaliculi have no wall of their own, but are formed as channels between adjacent liver cells, the plasmalemmata of which function as their linings (see also Fig. 342). Injection specimen (bile canaliculi: black; sinusoids: red). Magnification 380×.

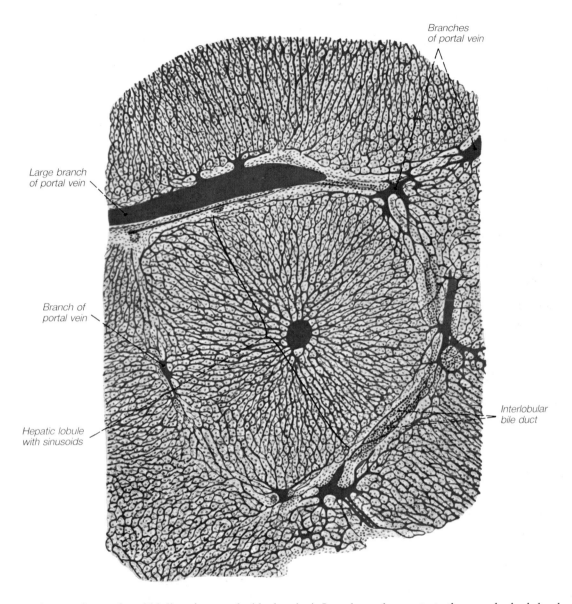

Branches of portal vein

Large branch of portal vein

Branch of portal vein

Hepatic lobule with sinusoids

Interlobular bile duct

Fig. 339. Injection specimen of a rabbit liver (camera lucida drawing). In order to demonstrate the vascular bed clearly, the organ has been perfused through the portal vein with a colored (Berlin blue) gelatin solution. Sometimes double injection, via both the portal and hepatic veins, is employed to delineate the two venous systems of the liver by different colors, the central veins forming the origin of the hepatic venous system. Borax-carmine staining. Magnification 54×.

Liver – Electron microscopy

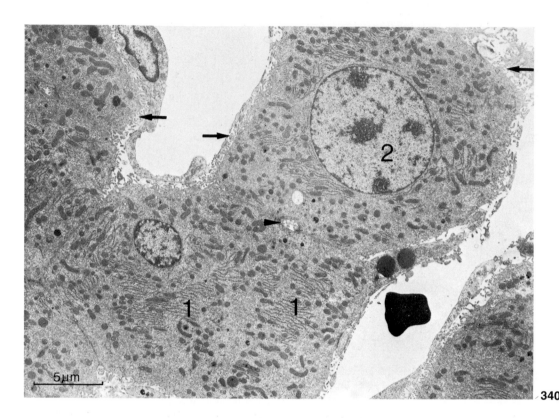

340

Fig. 340. Low-power electron micrograph of a rat liver illustrating two sinusoids together with adjoining hepatic cells (= hepatocytes). These cells are characterized by an abundance of mitochondria and regular stacks of rough endoplasmic reticulum (**1**). Towards the space of Disse, the cell surface is covered by closely spaced irregular microvilli (→) and other microvilli project into the bile canaliculus (►). **2** Nucleus of a hepatocyte. Magnification 3,500 ×.

Fig. 341. Transverse section through a rat liver sinusoid with a lymphocyte in its lumen. The extremely attenuated endothelium appears for the most part as a row of separate tiny cytoplasmic profiles and only occasionally forms a continuous cell layer over short distances (**1**). Note the large number of microvilli projecting from the hepatocytes into the space of Disse. Magnification 14,000 ×.

Fig. 342. Three hepatocytes bordering on a bile canaliculus (✳) that has no separate wall of its own. A few irregular microvilli project into the canalicular lumen. One of the liver cells clearly shows part of its nucleus (**1**), a regularly arranged rough ER (**2**), numerous mitochondria and glycogen particles (**3**). Magnification 14,000 ×.

156

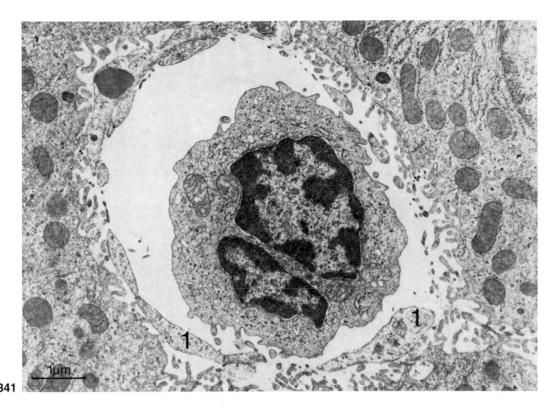

341

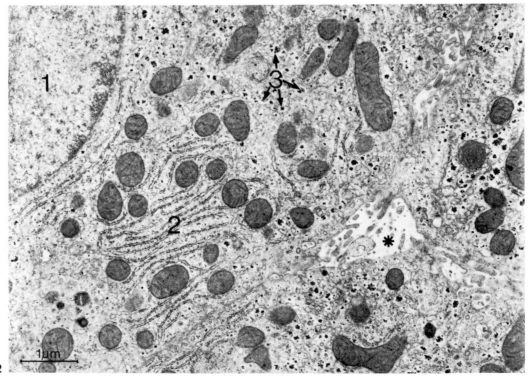

342

Digestive system – Pancreas

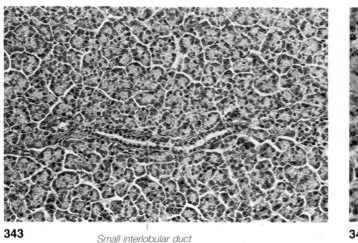

343

Small interlobular duct

Fig. 343. Exocrine portion of a human pancreas with part of a narrow interlobular duct. Despite the absence of islets of Langerhans, this specimen is still readily identifiable as pancreas and distinguishable from the other serous glands (for this see Figs. 307–309 and Table 12). Mallory-azan staining. Magnification 150×.

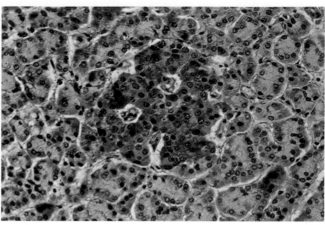

344

Fig. 344. Dog pancreatic islet with the β-granules selectively stained by chromium hematoxylin. With this technique A- and B-cells are distinguishable by their respective red and blue staining and their relative proportions can be measured. Chromium hematoxylin-phloxine staining. Magnification 280×.

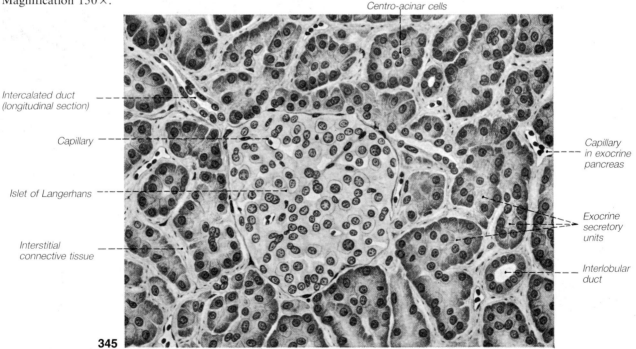

Centro-acinar cells

Intercalated duct (longitudinal section)

Capillary

Islet of Langerhans

Interstitial connective tissue

Capillary in exocrine pancreas

Exocrine secretory units

Interlobular duct

345

Fig. 345. Higher magnification shows the basophilic material found in the basal zones of the exocrine secretory cells, the light microscopic equivalent (ergastoplasm) of the RER (camera lucida drawing). The "centro-acinar" cells are a reflection of the deep invagination of the secretory units by the extremely narrow intercalated ducts, the duct lining cells thus apparently lying within the serous acini. Centro-acinar cells are of only limited value for identification purposes, because inexperienced microscopists have difficulties in picking out these morphological features. Islets of Langerhans are best found at magnifications where their paler staining shows them as rounded lighter areas within the exocrine glandular tissue. See Figure 344 for islet cell types and Figures 29, 31 and 308 for other structural details. H & E staining. Magnification 500×.

158

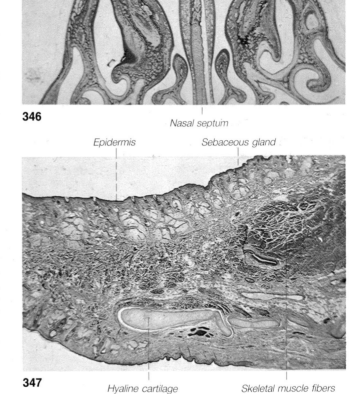

346

Olfactory bulb

Nasal septum

Fig. 346. Frontal section through the upper parts of a cat nasal cavity which, as in other species with a highly developed olfactory sense, has a much more elaborate system of conchae than that found in man. Note the cross-sectioned olfactory bulbs at the top of the micrograph. Mallory-azan staining. Magnification 10×.

Epidermis   *Sebaceous gland*

347

Hyaline cartilage   *Skeletal muscle fibers*

Fig. 347. Sections of the nasal ala are characterized by an outer covering of skin with sebaceous glands but no hairs and an inner surface lined similarly but showing occasionally thick hairs (= vibrissae). Other parts of the inner surface further inside and away from the hairs may be lined by a respiratory epithelium. The central core is composed of both hyaline cartilage and skeletal muscle fibers in varying proportions. See Table 11 for identifying characteristics. Mallory-azan staining. Magnification 10×.

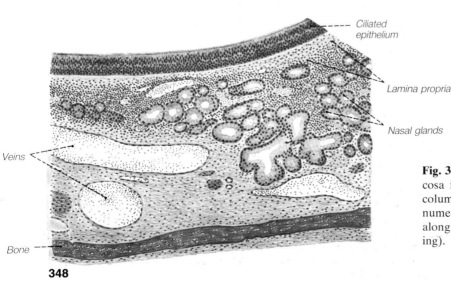

Ciliated epithelium

Lamina propria

Nasal glands

Veins

Bone

348

Fig. 348. The respiratory region of the nasal mucosa is characterized by a pseudostratified ciliated columnar epithelium and a lamina propria containing numerous tubulo-acinar (serous and mucous) glands along with many large veins (camera lucida drawing). H & E staining. Magnification 110×.

159

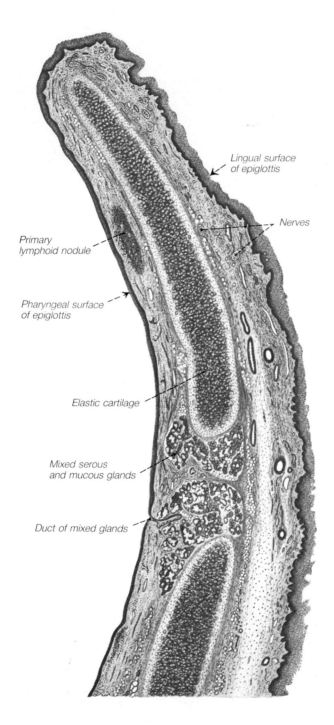

Lingual surface
of epiglottis

Nerves

Primary
lymphoid nodule

Pharyngeal surface
of epiglottis

Elastic cartilage

Mixed serous
and mucous glands

Duct of mixed glands

Fig. 349. Longitudinal section through a human epiglottis, the surfaces of which consist of a stratified noncornified squamous epithelium of different height (camera lucida drawing). The junction with the respiratory epithelium never occurs at the apex of the epiglottis and, as in this specimen, is often so low down as not to be included in the preparation. The main component of the central tissue core is an elastic cartilage. For further identifying characteristics, see Table 11. H & E staining. Magnification 4.5 ×.

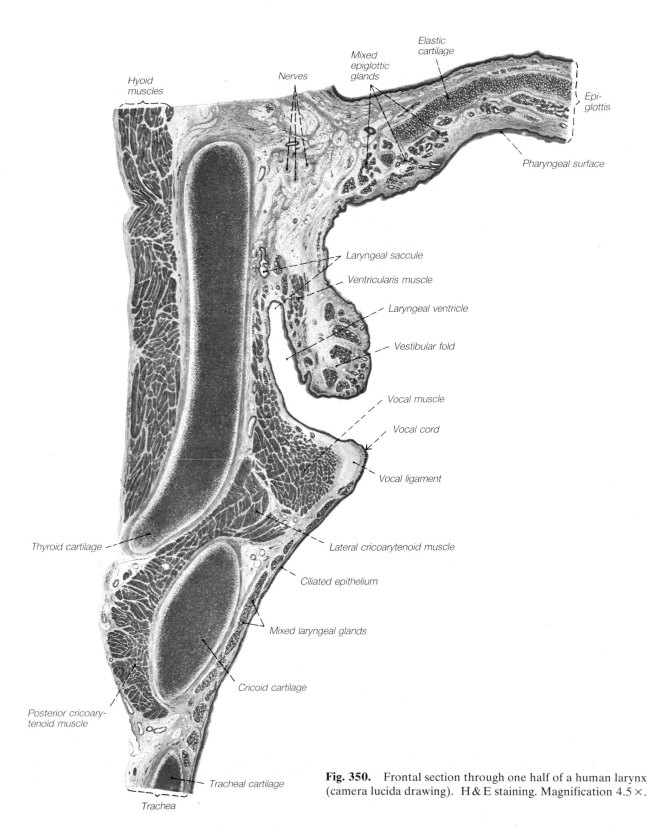

Hyoid
muscles

Nerves

Mixed
epiglottic
glands

Elastic
cartilage

Epi-
glottis

Pharyngeal surface

Laryngeal saccule

Ventricularis muscle

Laryngeal ventricle

Vestibular fold

Vocal muscle

Vocal cord

Vocal ligament

Lateral cricoarytenoid muscle

Ciliated epithelium

Mixed laryngeal glands

Thyroid cartilage

Cricoid cartilage

Posterior cricoary-
tenoid muscle

Tracheal cartilage

Trachea

Fig. 350. Frontal section through one half of a human larynx
(camera lucida drawing). H & E staining. Magnification 4.5 ×.

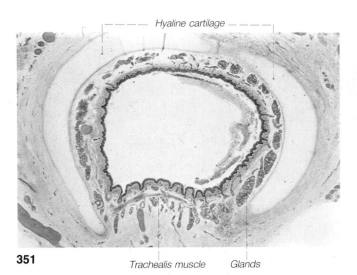

351

Hyaline cartilage

Trachealis muscle   Glands

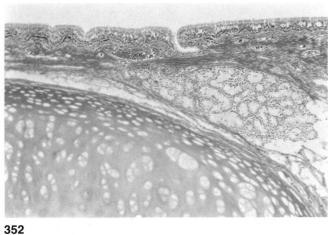

352

Fig. 351. Cross-section through a human fetal trachea, already showing all the structural characteristics of the fully developed state. The apparent variation in width of the C-shaped hyaline cartilage is the result of a slightly oblique section. Note the large number of small glands in the lamina propria and the trachealis muscle crossing the paries membranaceus (posterior part of the wall of the treachea). H & E staining. Magnification 14×.

Fig. 352. Longitudinal section through an adult trachea showing its mucosa made up of a ciliated pseudostratified columnar (respiratory) epithelium with an underlying fibrous lamina propria. The sero-mucous glands tend to be located in the spaces between successive hyaline cartilages. Mallory-azan staining. Magnification 62.5×.

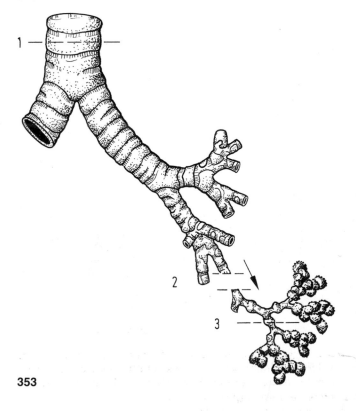

353

Fig. 353. Highly-simplified diagram of the trachea and its ramifications. Because of the restricted space, the large number of intrapulmonary bronchi (located between levels "2" and "3") have been omitted. Sections through the levels "1", "2" and "3" are represented by Figures 351, 354 a and 355, respectively.

162

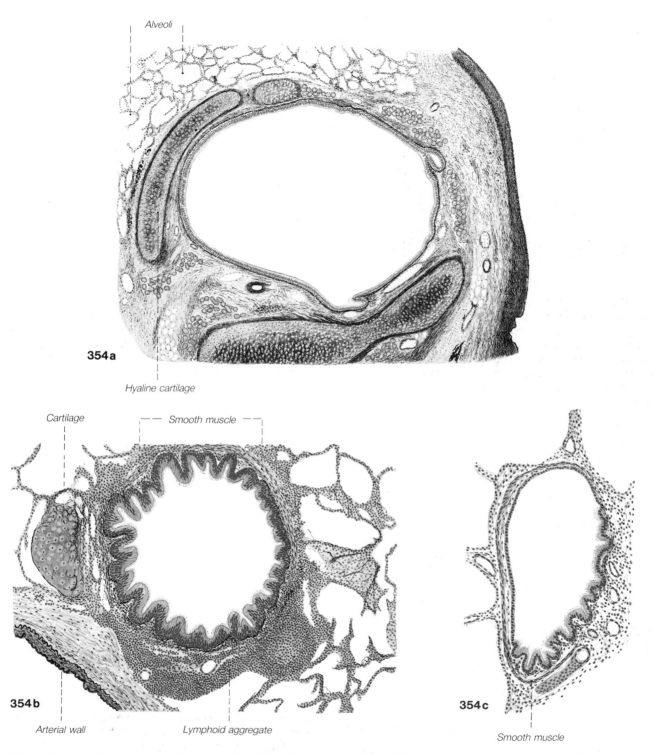

Alveoli

354a

Hyaline cartilage

Cartilage   *Smooth muscle*

354b

Arterial wall   *Lymphoid aggregate*

354c

Smooth muscle

Fig. 354. Cross-sections through different parts of the intrapulmonary bronchial tree (camera lucida drawings). Elastic and nuclear fast red staining. Magnification 30× (354a) and 60× (354b,c).
a) Small bronchus with large amounts of hyaline cartilage in its wall.
b) Terminal branch of a bronchus showing little cartilage and a lymphoid tissue aggregate.
c) Bronchiole devoid of cartilage but with obliquely and circularly oriented smooth muscle.

163

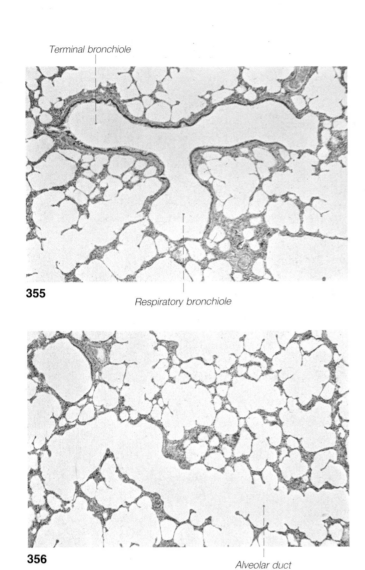

Terminal bronchiole

355

Respiratory bronchiole

356

Alveolar duct

Remnants of epithelium

357

358

Fig. 355. The point of branching of a terminal bronchiole into two respiratory bronchioles, the apparent blind endings of which are due to the plane of section. Note how the respiratory epithelium ends abruptly at the origins of the respiratory bronchioles. H & E staining. Magnification 38 ×.

Fig. 356. Longitudinal section through a respiratory bronchiole continuing into an alveolar duct (right side of the micrograph). There is a cross-sectioned terminal bronchiole in the upper left corner (human lung). H & E staining. Magnification 38 ×.

Fig. 357. Close-up of the site of transition shown in the preceding micrograph. Because of the large number of alveolar outpouchings, the wall of the alveolar duct seems discontinuous, apparently consisting of occasional short runs of epithelium underlain by smooth muscle bundles. H & E staining. Magnification 96 ×.

Fig. 358. Alveoli stained specifically for elastic fibers. In routine sections the complex three-dimensional network formed by these fibers is missed. They can, however, be visualized in thick sections by judicious use of the fine focus adjustment of the microscope (canine lung). Orcein staining. Magnification 96 ×.

Bronchus *Hyaline cartilage*

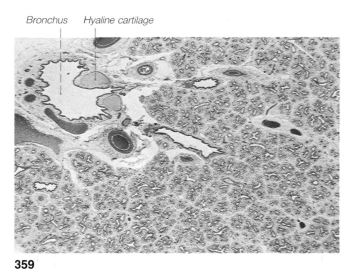

359

Mesenchymal interstitial connective tissue

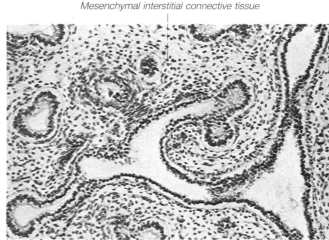

360

Fig. 359. Because it is an epithelial derivative the fetal lung at certain stages of its development consists of epithelially lined tubular cavities that show numerous dichotomous branches equipped with acinar endings. The fetal lung thus closely resembles certain glands with which it is easily confused (see Figs. 418–421 and Table 14). Mallory-azan staining. Magnification 38×.

Fig. 360. At a higher magnification the homogeneity of the lining of the cavities of the fetal lung is apparent and indicates its immaturity. In addition the mesenchymal nature of the interstitial connective tissue is shown by its high cellularity. Mallory-azan staining. Magnification 150×.

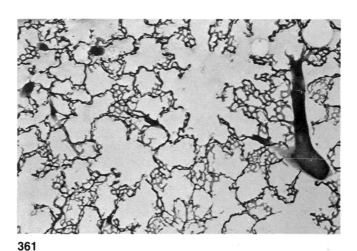

361

Fig. 361. The relatively narrow lung capillaries are only identified with certainty in routine preparations when they contain red cells. Only when they are artificially filled with a colored gelatin solution does the density of the capillaries and their three-dimensional basket-like arrangement around the alveoli become obvious (cat lung). Injection with Berlin blue gelatin through the pulmonary artery, no counterstaining. Magnification 95×.

Fig. 362. 1 μm thick plastic section of a cat lung in which the high capillary density is apparent even without the aid of injected solutions. This specimen also demonstrates the delicate nature of the air-blood barrier that is illustrated even better in the following electron micrographs. Methylene blue-azure II staining. Magnification 960×.

Capillary

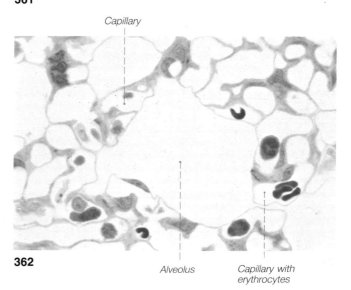

362

Alveolus   *Capillary with erythrocytes*

165

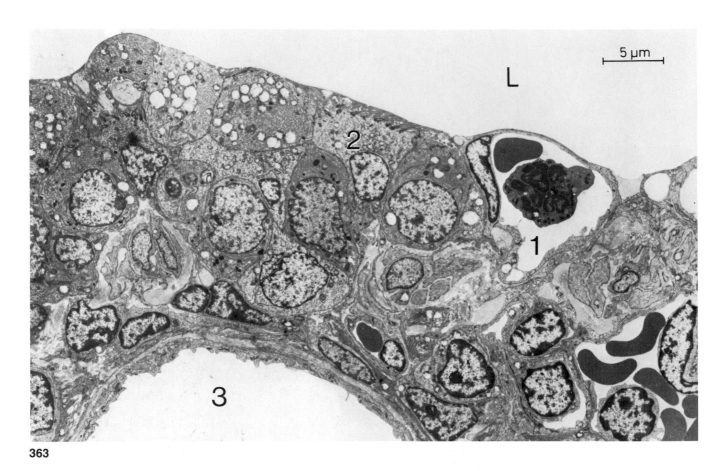

363

Fig. 363. Low-power electron micrograph from rabbit lung illustrating parts of an obliquely sectioned respiratory bronchiole with a capillary (**1**) bulging into its lumen (L). The lining simple epithelium is composed of different types of cells one of which is ciliated (**2**). A segment of a smaller branch (**3** arterial lumen) of the pulmonary artery, the arborizations of which usually accompany the bronchiolar ramifications, is seen in the lower part of this micrograph. Magnification 2,200 ×.

Fig. 364. Low-power electron micrograph of rabbit pulmonary alveolus (**1**) with its closely adjoining capillaries (**2**). Note the extreme attenuation of the blood-air barrier (→), which is shown to a better advantage at the right margin of this figure. This high-power electron micrograph illustrates that the barrier consists of two delicate cellular layers, the alveolar epithelium (alveolar type I cells: at the left side) and the intensely vesiculated capillary endothelium (at the right side). Both are separated by a narrow interstitial space which contains the fused epithelial and endothelial basal laminae resulting in a single lamina densa flanked on either side by a lamina rara. Magnifications 2,000 × and 45,000 ×, respectively.

Fig. 365 a). Part of an interstitial septum from rabbit lung displays small profile of alveolar type II cell (**1**) together with extracellular so-called tubular myelin (✳). These type II cells (= great alveolar cells) produce and secrete a material rich in phospholipids known as surfactant, which shows as thin parallel or concentric lamellae (►) within membrane-bound cavities. Exocytosed surfactant (→) is seen on the alveolar surface. **2** Capillary lumen; **3** Arteriolar lumina. Magnification 5,500 ×.

b) Close-up of the tubular myelin (✳) illustrates the orderly array of this lipidic material. To the left is a segment of a small arteriole. **L** Arteriolar lumen. Magnification 22,000 ×.

166

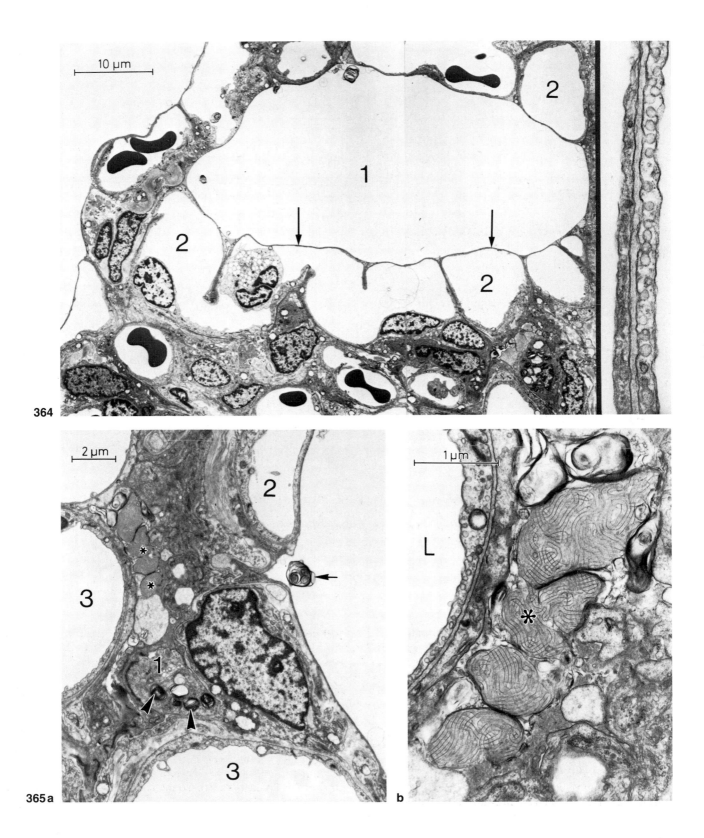

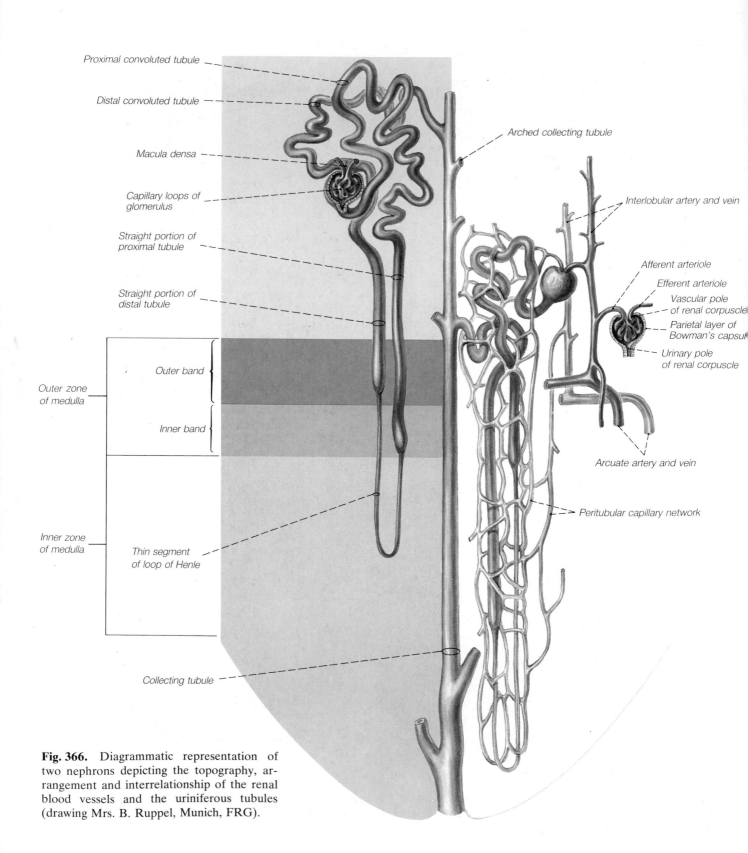

Proximal convoluted tubule

Distal convoluted tubule

Macula densa

Capillary loops of glomerulus

Straight portion of proximal tubule

Straight portion of distal tubule

Outer zone of medulla

Outer band

Inner band

Inner zone of medulla

Thin segment of loop of Henle

Collecting tubule

Arched collecting tubule

Interlobular artery and vein

Afferent arteriole

Efferent arteriole

Vascular pole of renal corpuscle

Parietal layer of Bowman's capsule

Urinary pole of renal corpuscle

Arcuate artery and vein

Peritubular capillary network

Fig. 366. Diagrammatic representation of two nephrons depicting the topography, arrangement and interrelationship of the renal blood vessels and the uriniferous tubules (drawing Mrs. B. Ruppel, Munich, FRG).

168

Glomerulus with afferent and efferent arteriole originating from radiating interlobular artery

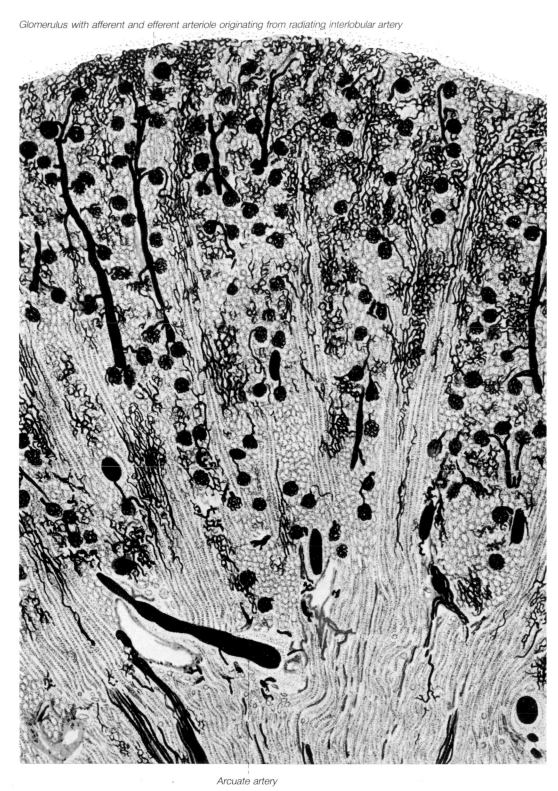

Arcuate artery

Fig. 367. Drawing of an injection specimen of human kidney. The vascular system has been filled via the renal artery with a colored (by Berlin blue) gelatin solution which has passed the glomeruli and thence the peritubular capillary network but it did not reach the venous outflow channels. Staining with nuclear fast red. Magnification 20×.

169

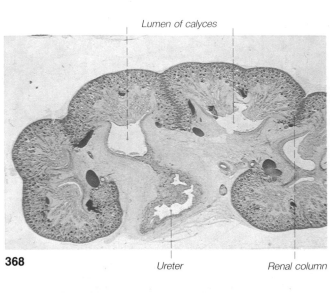

368
Lumen of calyces

Ureter   Renal column

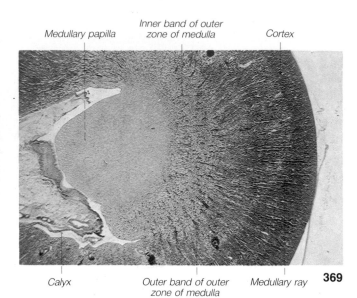

Inner band of outer
Medullary papilla   zone of medulla   Cortex

Calyx   Outer band of outer   Medullary ray   **369**
zone of medulla

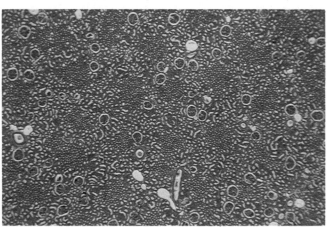

370
Glomerulus surrounded   Medullary rays (cross section)
by cortical labyrinth

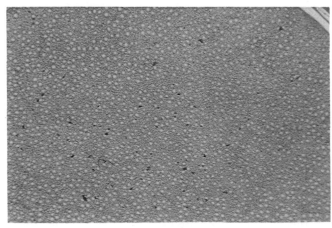

371

Fig. 368. Longitudinal section bisecting a human fetal kidney (18 cm crown-rump length) clearly showing the subdivision of the organ into lobes each of which possesses a medullary pyramid and thus one minor calyx. The renal parenchyma partly surrounds a cavity (= renal sinus) that contains the renal pelvis with its major and minor ramifications (= calyces) and the larger branches of the renal arteries, veins, lymphatics and nerves. In this specimen the major constituent of the sinus is connective tissue. Mallory-azan staining. Magnification 10×.

Fig. 369. Low-power view of a cross-sectioned rabbit kidney. The darker staining superficial parenchyma is the cortex, whose outermost layer is most intensely colored. The deeper paler region is the medulla subdivided into different zones – an innermost portion, the papilla, staining only poorly and covered by an inner and outer medullary zone (cf. Fig. 366). The outer medullary zone continues into the cortex in the form of radiating strands (= medullary rays), so that the border between these two layers is indistinct. Mallory-azan staining. Magnification 10×.

Fig. 370. In a tangential section through the renal cortex (man) its subdivision by the medullary rays is clearly seen. These mainly consist of the straight portions of the proximal and distal tubules and are surrounded by areas known as the cortical labyrinth containing the convoluted tubules and renal corpuscles. H&E staining. Magnification 24×.

Fig. 371. Low-power view of a cross-sectioned renal papilla (man) whose most characteristic features at such a low magnification are the numerous uniform and regularly spaced lumina, each of which corresponds to a transverse section of a collecting tubule (compare with Fig. 379). H&E staining. Magnification 24×.

Afferent arteriole   Macula densa

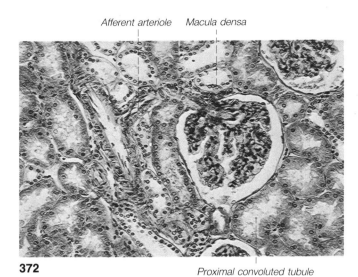

372   *Proximal convoluted tubule*

Macula densa

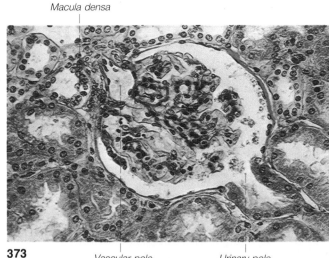

373   *Vascular pole*   *Urinary pole*

Distal convoluted tubule   *Proximal convoluted tubule*

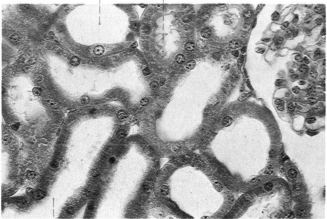

Proximal convoluted tubule   **374**

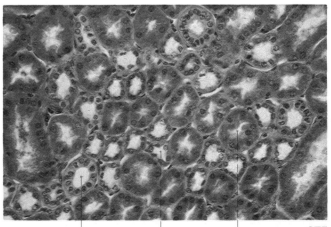

Collecting tubule   *Distal tubule*   *Proximal tubule*   **375**
                        (straight portion)   *(straight portion)*

Fig. 372. Coming from an obliquely oriented interlobular artery (in the left side of the micrograph) is an afferent arteriole that can be followed into the vascular pole of the renal corpuscle. Immediately above the corpuscle is a cross-section of a distal convoluted tubule with the macula densa lying adjacent to Bowman's capsule (human kidney). Mallory-azan staining. Magnification 150×.

Fig. 373. Human renal corpuscle with urinary and vascular poles. At the urinary pole the flattened parietal layer of Bowman's capsule is continuous with the taller epithelium of the proximal convoluted tubule. The visceral layer of Bowman's capsule consists of podocytes that encircle the glomerular capillaries with their processes. Note the prominent macula densa adjacent to the vascular pole. The tubular profiles surrounding the glomerulus belong to proximal and distal convoluted tubules (for their differentiation, see the next micrograph). Mallory-azan staining. Magnification 240×.

Fig. 374. The prominent brush border found in the proximal convoluted tubules allows their differentiation from the corresponding segments of the distal tubules, the latter also showing a less acidophilic cytoplasm. In some areas, e.g., the upper arrowed proximal tubule, the basal striations of the proximal convoluted tubules are visible (cf. Figs. 28 and 39). Mallory-azan staining. Magnification 380×.

Fig. 375. A higher magnification of a medullary ray clearly shows the differences between the proximal and distal segments of the uriniferous tubules. In the proximal tubules, the taller and deeper staining (more acidophilic) epithelium bulging into the lumen together with the brush border, produces an irregular poorly-defined luminal outline. In comparison, the lumina of the distal tubules with their lower epithelium appear larger and their outlines more clear-cut. Thus the ratio between epithelial height and tubular lumen is in favor of the latter in the distal segments. This feature is even more pronounced in the collecting tubules with their increased luminal diameters and their taller epithelium (tangential section through human renal cortex, cf. Figs. 376, 377). H & E staining. Magnification 240×.

171

Collecting tubule | Thick limb of Henle's loop

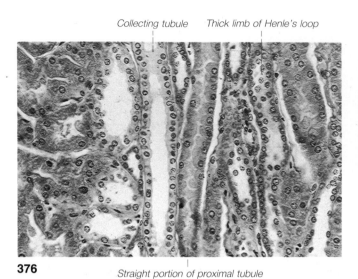

376
Straight portion of proximal tubule

Collecting tubule

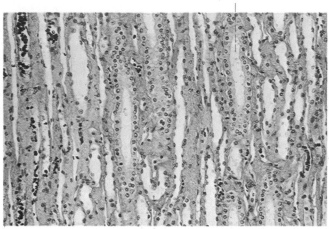

377
Bend of Henle's loop

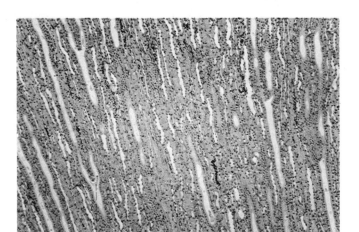

378
Fusion of collecting tubules

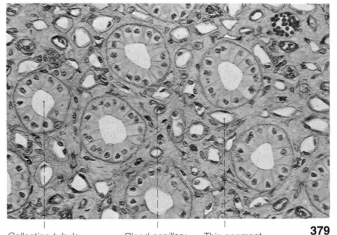

Collecting tubule | Blood capillary | Thin segment of Henle's loop

379

Fig. 376. Longitudinal section of a medullary ray (human kidney) with, at the left, parts of the adjacent cortical labyrinth. In the straight portion of the proximal tubule, the bulging of the epithelial cells and consequent luminal narrowing is clearly displayed. The collecting tubule, in contrast, has a wide lumen bordered by an even epithelial surface. The straight portion of the distal segment (to the right) is sectioned tangentially and thus can be differentiated from its proximal counterpart by the greater number of nuclei it contains. Mallory-azan staining. Magnification 240×.

Fig. 377. Longitudinal section through the outer medullary zone (human kidney) in which the thin segments of Henle's loop, which are lined by an extremely low epithelium, are prominent. Their descending and ascending limbs join in a U-shaped apex that is always directed toward the tip of the medullary papillae. Mallory-azan staining. Magnification 150×.

Fig. 378. Longitudinal section through the outer medullary zone (human kidney) with numerous longitudinally sectioned collecting tubules that gradually join, finally forming the papillary ducts opening onto the apex of the papilla. Note the numerous profiles of thin segments of Henle's loops lying between the collecting tubules which they parallel. Mallory-azan staining. Magnification 60×.

Fig. 379. In a cross-sectioned renal papilla (human kidney) the profiles of the collecting tubules are particularly prominent because of their large lumina and tall columnar epithelium (a low-power view is shown in Fig. 371). Running parallel are thin segments of Henle's loops and blood capillaries. The thin segments have a slightly higher epithelium with nuclei bulging into the lumen, while capillaries are smaller, with nuclei only rarely seen in cross-sections, and contain red blood cells. H & E staining. Magnification 240×.

Proximal convoluted tubule   Efferent arteriole

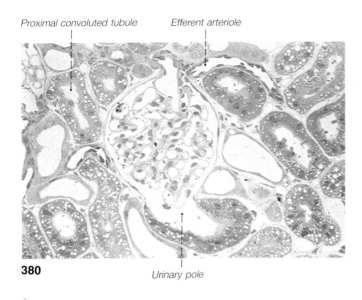

380   Urinary pole

Capsular space   Brush border

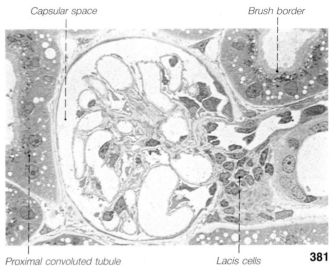

Proximal convoluted tubule   Lacis cells   **381**

    Brush border   Urinary pole

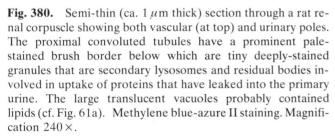

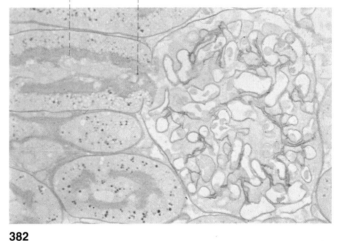

382

Fig. 380. Semi-thin (ca. 1 µm thick) section through a rat renal corpuscle showing both vascular (at top) and urinary poles. The proximal convoluted tubules have a prominent pale-stained brush border below which are tiny deeply-stained granules that are secondary lysosomes and residual bodies involved in uptake of proteins that have leaked into the primary urine. The large translucent vacuoles probably contained lipids (cf. Fig. 61a). Methylene blue-azure II staining. Magnification 240×.

Fig. 381. Renal corpuscle (rat) with vascular pole leading to efferent arteriole on the right. Below the vascular pole are a group of extraglomerular mesangial cells (also called lacis or Goormaghtigh cells) that belong to the juxtaglomerular apparatus and are wedged between the afferent and efferent arterioles. To the right of these cells is part of a macula densa. (The epithelioid juxtaglomerular or "Polkissen" cells are not represented in this semi-thin section). Methylene blue-azure II staining. Magnification 600×.

Fig. 382. Renal corpuscle of a rat in semi-thin section. The basal laminae of the glomerulus and renal tubules are shown as a delicate violet band by a modified PAS technique. Note also the PAS-positive reaction of the brush border and fine intracytoplasmic granules in the proximal tubules. Modified PAS staining. Magnification 480× (specimen courtesy of Prof. P. Böck, Vienna).

Fig. 383. Renal cortex of a rat with prominent "labeling" of the convoluted parts of the proximal tubules by the uptake and storage of the vital dye trypan blue. Nuclear fast red staining. Magnification 150×.

Renal capsule

383   Glomerulus

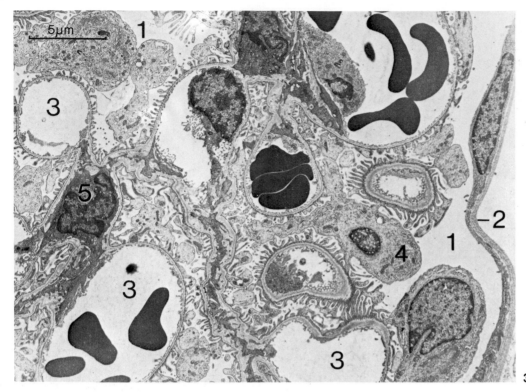

384

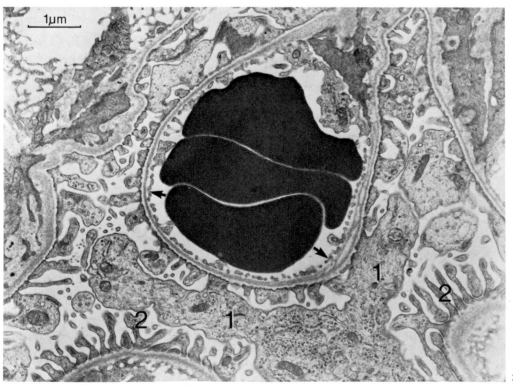

385

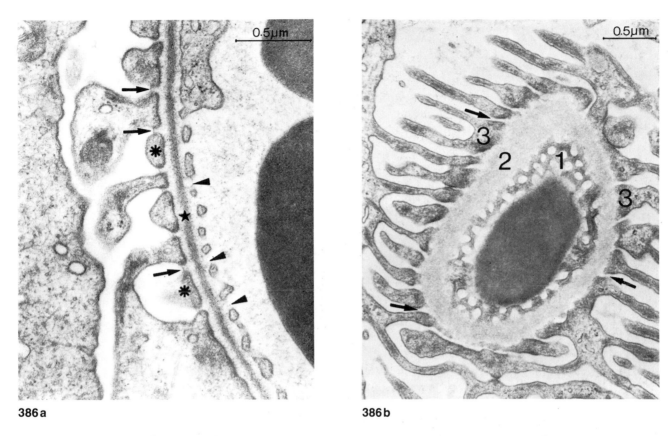

386 a   386 b

Fig. 386 a).   Transverse section through a glomerular capillary to demonstrate the structures that constitute the filtration barrier. Due to the abundance of pores or fenestrae (►) which perforate it, the endothelium usually appears as a row of unconnected cytoplasmic islets. The lamina densa (★) of the basal lamina is particularly thick (50–60 nm) in the glomerulus and acts as a coarse barrier for high molecular weight substances. The main filtration barrier is a delicate membrane, the slit membrane (→), that bridges the narrow cleft (= slit pores) between the foot processes (＊). Parts of an erythrocyte are seen in the capillary lumen. Magnification 40,000 ×.

b)   A tangential section of a glomerular capillary better illustrates the sieve-like structure of the endothelium (**1**) and the close investment of the basal lamina (**2**) by numerous interdigitating podocyte foot processes (**3**) separated by narrow (20–40 nm) intercellular clefts or slit pores (→). Magnification 27,000 ×.

Fig. 384.   Low-power electron micrograph illustrating part of a rat renal corpuscle with its capsular space (**1**), the parietal layer of Bowman's capsule (**2**) and several profiles of glomerular capillaries (**3**). Between the capillaries are two cell types, podocytes (**4**) and the more electron-dense mesangial cells (**5**). Magnification 4,000 ×.

Fig. 385.   A higher magnification of the preceding micrograph clearly reveals the large number of pores (→) crossing the endothelium. It also illustrates the complex system of podocyte cytoplasmic extensions subdivided into large primary (**1**) and slender secondary (**2**) processes, the latter called foot processes or pedicles. The primary processes (**1**) belong to the podocyte labeled "4" in the preceding micrograph. Magnification 14,000 ×.

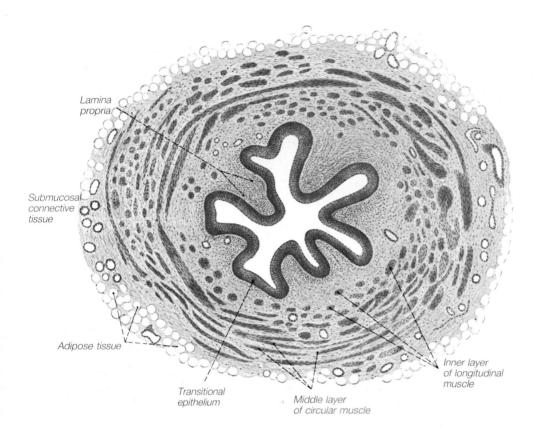

Lamina propria

Submucosal connective tissue

Adipose tissue

Transitional epithelium

Middle layer of circular muscle

Inner layer of longitudinal muscle

Fig. 387. Transverse section of a human ureter, the lumen narrowed to a star-shaped outline by contraction of the muscularis (see also Table 15). The muscularis consists of inner longitudinal, middle circular and less-developed outer longitudinal layers that are continuous with each other and thus poorly defined. This is explained by the fact that the smooth muscle bundles form continuous strands wound spirally around the long axis of the ureter (camera lucida drawing). H&E staining. Magnification 30×.

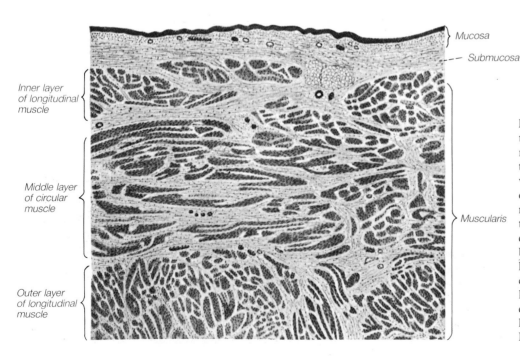

Inner layer of longitudinal muscle

Middle layer of circular muscle

Outer layer of longitudinal muscle

Mucosa

Submucosa

Muscularis

Fig. 388. The basic organization of the muscularis of the human urinary bladder is similar to that of the ureter with the individual muscle bundles being parts of continuous spirally-wound muscular strands. Because of this, they are oriented not in an exact circular or longitudinal fashion, but more or less obliquely to the long axis of the bladder. Considerable distension of the bladder has resulted in thinning of the epithelium (cf. Fig. 390, camera lucida drawing). H&E staining. Magnification 18×.

Transverse sections through ureter and urinary bladder (distended as well as contracted) from a baboon that are all shown with the same magnification (100 ×) to allow comparison of total wall thickness.

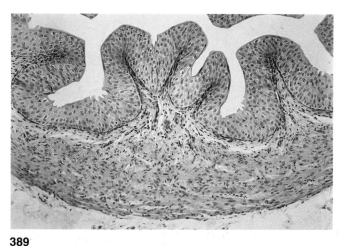

389

Fig. 389. Segment of a cross-sectioned ureter from a baboon with prominent mucosal folds and a thick (collapsed or compressed) transitional epithelium. The muscularis consists of interlacing strands of smooth muscle cells and lacks distinct lamination as seen in human ureter. H & E staining. Magnification 100 ×.

Epithelium   Bundle of smooth muscle cells

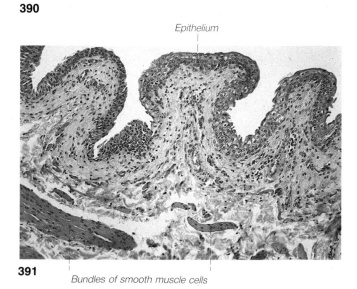

390

Fig. 390. Complete cross-section of a maximally dilated (passively stretched) urinary bladder from a baboon. Notice pronounced attenuation of both the transitional epithelium (its height is less than half of that seen in the contracted state) and the muscularis whose entire thickness is included in this micrograph. H & E staining. Magnification 100 ×.

Epithelium

Fig. 391. This micrograph shows a piece from the same urinary bladder as illustrated in the preceding figure, but the bladder has been allowed to contract. The mucosa is thrown into prominent folds covered by a thick transitional epithelium. Notice that in this case only the submucosa together with the innermost strands of the muscularis are included in this micrograph taken with the same magnification as that used in the preceding figure. H & E staining. Magnification 100 ×.

391

Bundles of smooth muscle cells

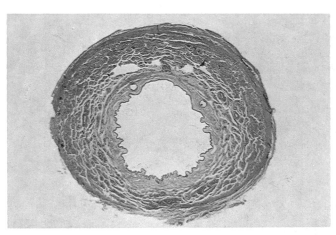

392

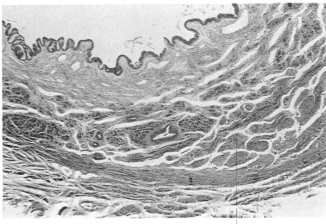

393   *Bundle of smooth muscle cells*

Artery

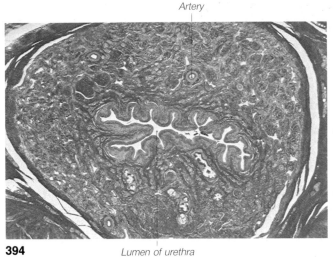

394   *Lumen of urethra*

Fig. 392. A cross-section of a human female urethra shows its rather wide lumen. The muscularis, consisting of small muscle bundles, is indistinct, although more pronounced towards the periphery. Mallory-azan staining. Magnification 10 ×.

Fig. 393. A higher magnification discloses the numerous veins in the lamina propria that assist in firm closure of the urethra. No glands of Littré are included in this section. The epithelium is stratified columnar (see Fig. 84 for details). Mallory-azan staining. Magnification 62 ×.

Fig. 394. Transverse section through the cavernous (spongy) portion of the male urethra, the identification of which is made easy by the surrounding mass of erectile tissue. H & E staining. Magnification 10 ×.

Lumen of urethra

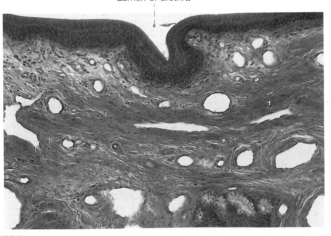

395

Fig. 395. This higher magnification shows that the epithelium is two- to three-layered and, because of the shape of the cells in the surface layer, columnar in type. H & E staining. Magnification 100 ×.

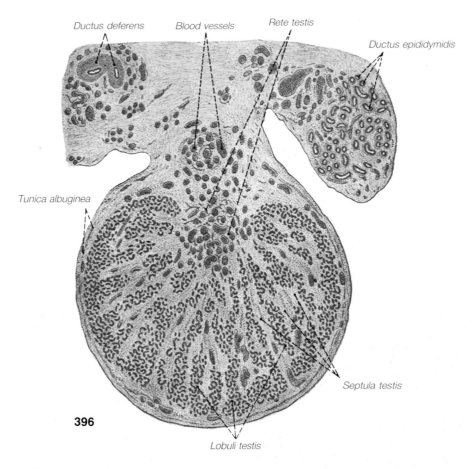

Ductus deferens   Blood vessels   Rete testis   Ductus epididymidis

Tunica albuginea

Septula testis

396

Lobuli testis

Fig. 396. Low-power view of an immature human testis. Radiating from the capsule (= tunica albuginea) towards the mediastinum are connective tissue septa (= septula testis) that divide the organ into lobules (= lobuli testis), each of which contains several intricately coiled tubules, the convoluted seminiferous tubules. These tubules empty through the rete testis located in the mediastinum into the ductuli efferentes in the head of the epididymis (camera lucida drawing). H & E staining. Magnification 16×.

Primordial germ cell

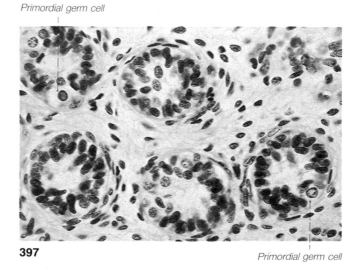

Fig. 397. The seminiferous tubules of this human fetal testis are predominantly solid (germinal) cords consisting of only two cell types, the prevailing one being the primitive Sertoli cells that stand out because of their closely-spaced deeply staining nuclei. The second type of cells are the primordial germ cells which migrate along the dorsal mesentery of the hindgut into the gonadal ridge. These cells are identified by 1) their large size, 2) their pale-staining cytoplasm and 3) their spherical nuclei. Mallory-azan staining. Magnification 380×.

397

Primordial germ cell

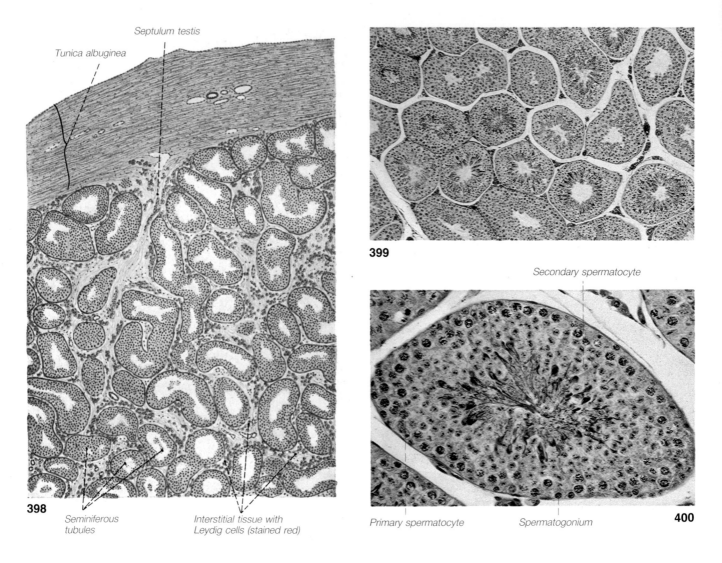

398

Tunica albuginea

Septulum testis

399

Secondary spermatocyte

Seminiferous tubules

Interstitial tissue with Leydig cells (stained red)

Primary spermatocyte

Spermatogonium

400

Fig. 398.   Peripheral part of a mature human testis. The testis is enclosed in a dense fibrous capsule (tunica albuginea), the outer surface of which is covered by the visceral layer (= epiorchium) of the tunica vaginalis. In the interstices between seminiferous tubules, the loosely aggregated and strongly acidophilic interstitial cells of Leydig can be seen (camera lucida drawing). H & E staining. Magnification 40×.

Fig. 399.   Low-power view of several seminiferous tubules from a rat testis. Such specimens are often used in histological courses since in rodents spermatogenic activity occurs in a wavelike fashion along the tubules. Because of this, different stages of spermatogenesis will prevail in different tubular cross-sections and the details of these stages are particularly clearly seen. Weigert's iron hematoxylin and benzo light Bordeaux staining. Magnification 60×.

Fig. 400.   Cross-sectioned seminiferous tubule from a rat testis. Although there are a few scattered spermatogonia, most of the epithelium consists of primary spermatocytes (recognized by their prominent chromatin) and their daughter cells, the secondary spermatocytes. The lumen of the tubule is packed with the tails of spermatozoa. Although the spermatozoal heads appear to lie deep within the germ cells, in actual fact groups (usually of eight) of them are enveloped by cytoplasmic processes of the Sertoli cells. Weigert's iron hematoxylin and benzo light Bordeaux staining. Magnification 240×.

Fig. 401. Cross-sectioned seminiferous convoluted tubule from human testis showing nearly all stages of spermatogenesis. Adjacent to the basement membrane are cells with spherical nuclei, the spermatogonia. On their inner aspect lie the primary spermatocytes that are larger, but that also have spherical nuclei.

The primary spermatocytes arise from the spermatogonia by a mitotic cell division followed by a growth period. Then, by the first maturation division, each primary spermatocyte produces two secondary spermatocytes (= prespermatids) that are half the size of the mother cell. Barely visible in this specimen are the spermatids that result from the second maturation division, but the arrow-shaped heads of the spermatozoa stand out as darkly stained structures. In the connective tissue interstices are groups of interstitial (Leydig) cells (for details, see Fig. 51). Mallory-azan staining. Magnification 240×.

Fig. 402. A higher magnification of the epithelial lining of a human seminiferous tubule to illustrate the nuclei of Sertoli cells. These differ from all the germ cells by always showing an indistinct chromatin but prominent nucleolus. Note the telophase of a spermatogonial mitotic division at the lower left margin of the tubule. Mallory-azan staining. Magnification 380×.

Fig. 403. Since diagnostic analysis of human spermatogenesis is routinely performed today on semi-thin plastic sections such a specimen from rat testis is shown here. Notice significantly enhanced cytological details as compared to the paraplast embedded material of the preceding figures. Thionine staining. Magnification 250×.

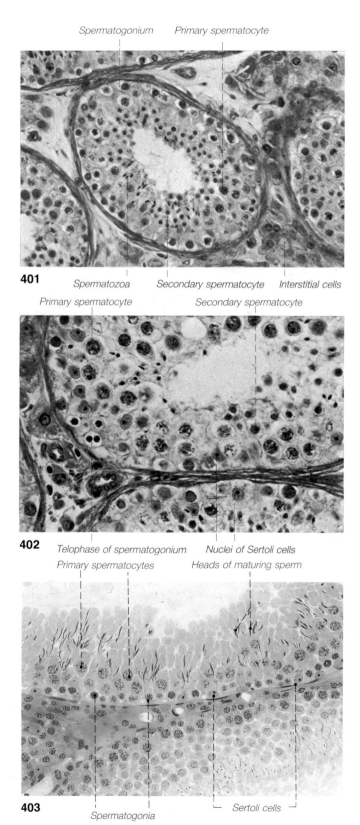

Spermatogonium   Primary spermatocyte

401   Spermatozoa   Secondary spermatocyte   Interstitial cells

Primary spermatocyte   Secondary spermatocyte

402   Telophase of spermatogonium   Nuclei of Sertoli cells

Primary spermatocytes   Heads of maturing sperm

403   Spermatogonia   Sertoli cells

181

Ductus epididymidis

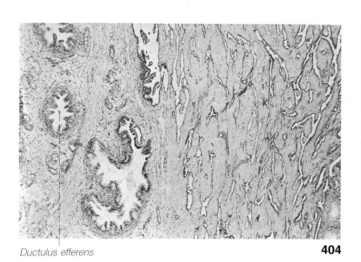

Ductulus efferens   **404**

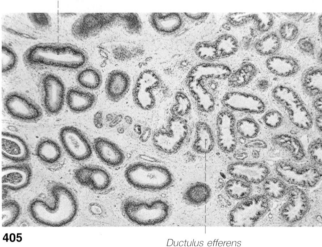

405

Ductulus efferens

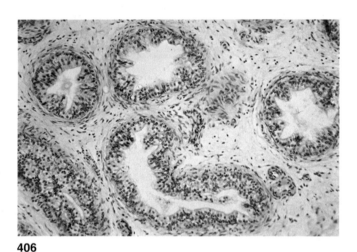

406

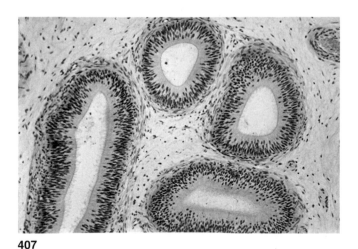

407

Fig. 404. Section through the testicular mediastinum (right side) and the adjacent head of a human epididymis. The richly-branched narrow anastomosing tubules in the mediastinum are the rete testis, the beginnings of the excretory duct system of the testis. They empty into the ductuli efferentes located within the head of the epididymis. H & E staining. Magnification 38 ×.

Fig. 405. Low-power view of a human epididymis illustrating the two types of ducts found in this organ. The tortuous ductuli efferentes (right side) are located in the head, while the even more convoluted ductus epididymidis occupies the body and tail. The lumina of the ductuli efferentes have a characteristic serrated outline which distinguishes these tubules from the ductus epididymidis with its even inner contour. H & E staining. Magnification 25 ×.

Fig. 406. At higher magnification it is obvious that both the number of layers and the height of the epithelial cells vary at quite regular intervals around the circumference of a ductulus efferens. Those parts projecting into the lumen consist of a pseudostratified or stratified columnar epithelium furnished with motile cilia, while the crypt-like depressions are lined by a non-ciliated pseudostratified cuboidal epithelium. The cilia are not visible at this magnification. H & E staining. Magnification 96 ×.

Fig. 407. The pseudostratified tall columnar epithelium of the ductus epididymidis is uniform in height and equipped with stereocilia, but these cell surface specializations are not visible at this magnification (for details, see Figs. 85 and 93). H & E staining. Magnification 96 ×.

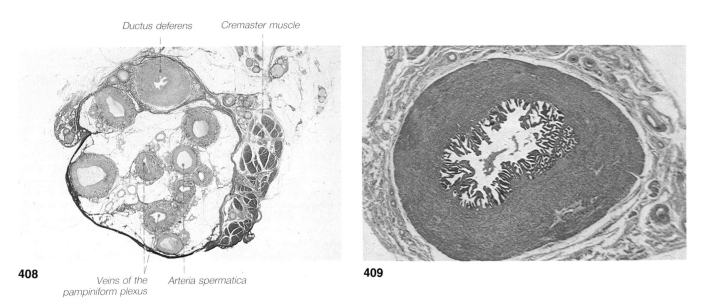

408

Ductus deferens   Cremaster muscle

Veins of the pampiniform plexus   Arteria spermatica

409

Fig. 408. Cross-section through a human spermatic cord containing the ductus deferens and numerous blood vessels. Although most of the vessels belong to the venous pampiniform plexus, veins in this region have a thick three-layered media and are thus easily mistaken for arteries. The cremaster muscle is seen at the right periphery of the cord. H & E staining. Magnification 7 ×.

Fig. 409. Transverse section through the ampulla of a human ductus deferens. In contrast to the ductus deferens proper, the epithelium here covers a complex network of anastomosing folds and the three layers of the muscularis are indistinct, the circular component predominating. The ampulla of the ductus deferens is sometimes confused with the seminal vesicle, but can be distinguished by 1) its narrow lumen, 2) its thicker muscularis and 3) its less-developed mucosal folds (cf. Figs. 411–413). H & E staining. Magnification 17 ×.

Fig. 410. Especially characteristic of the human ductus deferens is the thick muscularis subdivided into three layers. These layers represent continuous muscle strands that encircle the ductus in a spiral fashion. Since the inner and outer parts of the spiral are steep, while the middle portion is rather flat, the impression in cross-section is of outer longitudinal, middle circular and inner longitudinal muscle layers. The epithelium is pseudostratified columnar with stereocilia that stop at the end of the ductus. As in comparable tubes, e.g., the ureter, the lumen is stellate (see Table 15) because of muscular contraction (camera lucida drawing). H & E staining. Magnification 50 ×.

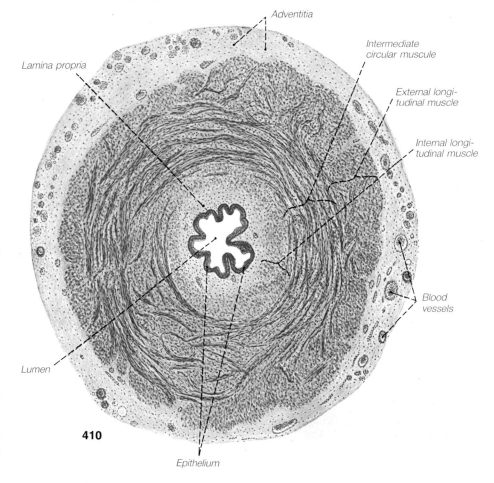

Adventitia

Intermediate circular muscle

External longitudinal muscle

Internal longitudinal muscle

Lamina propria

Blood vessels

Lumen

410

Epithelium

183

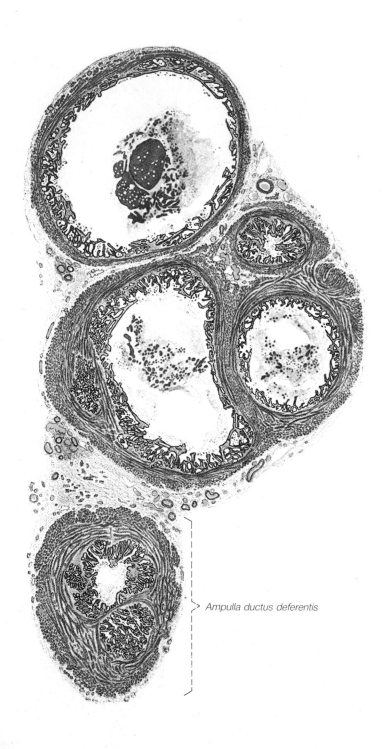

Ampulla ductus deferentis

Fig. 411. Low-power view of a seminal vesicle together with the ampulla of the ductus deferens, distinguished from one another by the size of the lumina and the thickness of the muscle coats (camera lucida drawing). Compare with Figures 409 and 412. H & E staining. Magnification 10×.

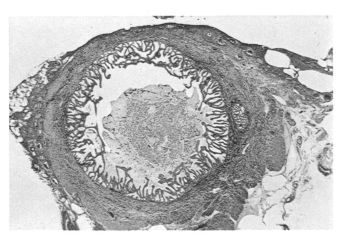

412

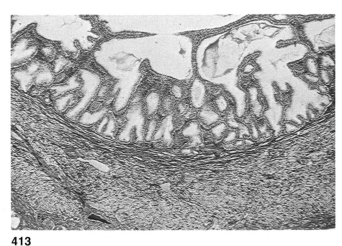

413

Fig. 412. Cross-section of a human seminal vesicle with its mucosa thrown into a characteristic complex pattern of interconnected folds. The muscularis consists mainly of obliquely and longitudinally oriented fiber bundles not arranged in definite layers. Differentiation from the ampulla of the ductus deferens is based on 1) the wider lumen, 2) the more elaborate mucosal folds and 3) the thinner muscularis. Mallory-azan staining. Magnification 17×.

Fig. 413. A higher magnification shows the filigree-like nature of the mucosa due to the numerous anastomoses between its folds. As in the gallbladder (see Fig. 327), this mucosa shows many irregular cavities lined by epithelium. The greater number of these cavities and the much thicker muscularis distinguishes this organ from the gallbladder. Mallory-azan staining. Magnification 48×.

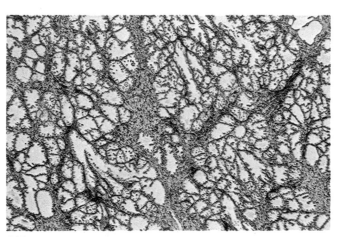

414

Fig. 414. Low-power view of the human prostate gland. Sections through this tubulo-alveolar gland show rather large irregular often-indented cavities between which excretory ducts are only rarely seen. This last feature discriminates the prostate from the lactating mammary gland with which it is often confused (see Figs. 418–421 and Table 14 for differentiation). Mallory-azan staining. Magnification 38×.

Fig. 415. At higher magnification it is seen that the columnar epithelium of the prostatic alveoli varies in height and is thrown into delicate folds that give the secretory elements a frill-like inner contour. A unique feature of the prostate gland is the vast number of interlacing smooth muscle bundles coursing within the connective tissue septa. Mallory-azan staining. Magnification 150×.

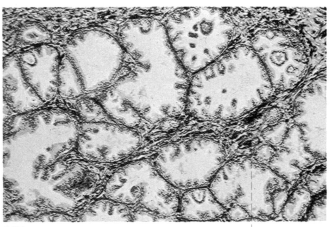

415

Smooth muscle

Penis

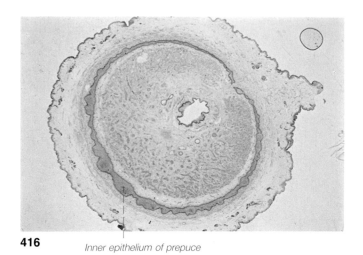

416

Inner epithelium of prepuce

Fig. 416. Cross-section through an infant glans penis at the level of the fossa navicularis. Because the inner epithelial lining of the prepuce is still "glued" to the covering epithelium of the glans, the glans itself is encircled by a solid epithelial glando-preputial lamella. In the vicinity of its external orifice, the urethra is lined by a stratified squamous noncornified epithelium. H & E staining (faded). Magnification 10×.

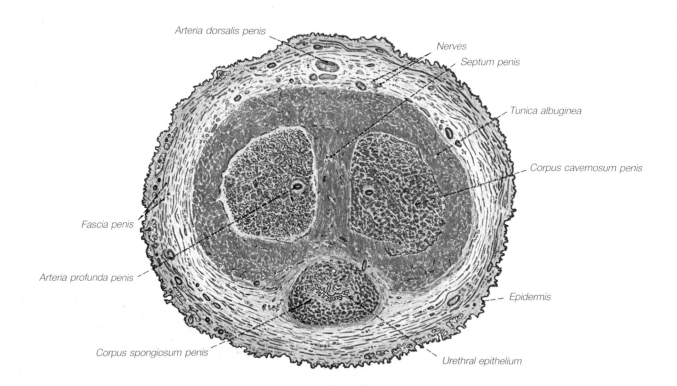

Arteria dorsalis penis

Nerves

Septum penis

Tunica albuginea

Corpus cavernosum penis

Fascia penis

Arteria profunda penis

Epidermis

Corpus spongiosum penis

Urethral epithelium

Fig. 417. Cross-section through the shaft of an adult human penis (camera lucida drawing). See Figs. 394 and 395 for details of the corpus spongiosum and the urethra it encloses. H & E staining. Magnification 4×.

186

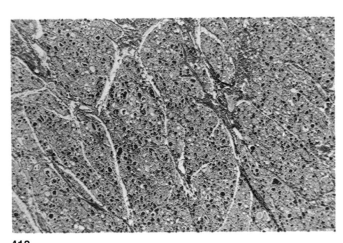

418

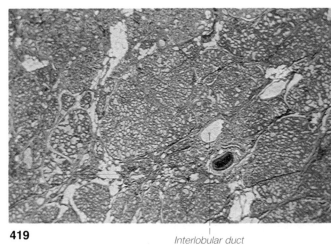

419

Interlobular duct

Bronchus

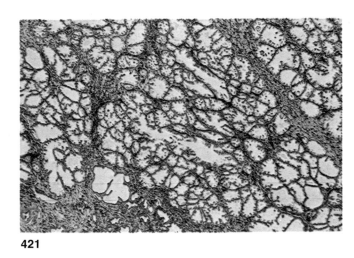

420

Figs. 418–421. When comparing sections of those alveolar glands that are often confused with each other – the thyroid (Fig. 418), prostate (Fig. 421) and lactating mammary gland (Fig. 419) – the prostate gland clearly differs from the two other glands by its lack of distinct lobular subdivisions and by the unique presence of smooth muscle cells in its connective tissue interstices. The lactating mammary gland is distinguished from the thyroid by its consistently large excretory ducts, whereas the thyroid has secretory units (= follicles) that vary considerably in size and in the amount of colloid they contain. The fetal lung (Fig. 420) is illustrated in this section because, like the glands, it arises as an epithelial sprout and thus shows a similar growth pattern. The fetal lung is often confused with an active mammary gland, particularly when the preparation has not first been examined with the lowest-power objective for its most typical feature, the bronchial primordia, identified by the hyaline cartilage in their walls (see also Fig. 359 and Table 14). A further characteristic of the fetal lung is its highly cellular and very loose connective tissue (cf. Fig. 360). All Figures: Mallory-azan staining. Magnification 38×.

421

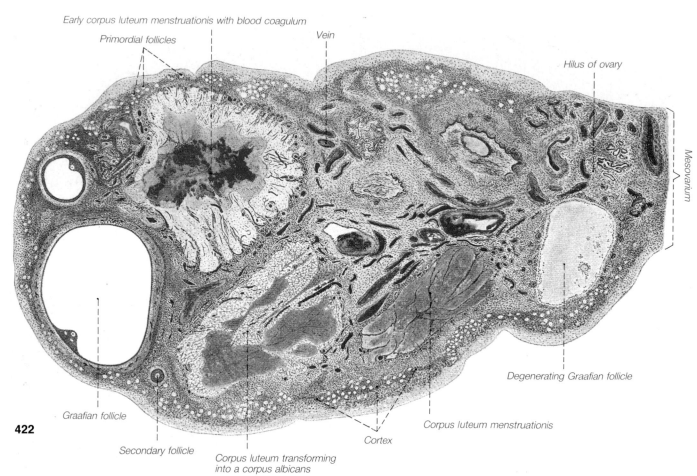

Early corpus luteum menstruationis with blood coagulum

Primordial follicles

Vein

Hilus of ovary

Mesovarium

Graafian follicle

Secondary follicle

Corpus luteum transforming into a corpus albicans

Cortex

Corpus luteum menstruationis

Degenerating Graafian follicle

422

Fig. 422. Complete transverse section of a human ovary in a partly schematic drawing made from a series of histologic specimens (after Patzelt: *Histologie*, 3rd ed., Urban & Schwarzenberg, Vienna 1948). In order to identify the various stages of development of ovarian follicles, suitable areas for study must first be selected by use of the lower-power objective. Since this can be difficult in human specimens, ovaries from laboratory animals are often shown in histology courses. H & E staining. Magnification 10 ×.

Nucleus of oocyte

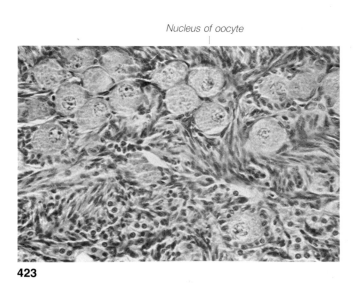

423

Fig. 423. Cortex of a cat ovary showing a number of primordial follicles, each of which consists of a primary oocyte, surrounded by a single layer of squamous or cuboidal epithelium, the follicular epithelium. Primordial follicles are occasionally confused with spinal ganglion cells (cf. Figs. 19, 523), particularly if the section is examined only at high magnification. H & E staining. Magnification 240 ×.

Primary follicles

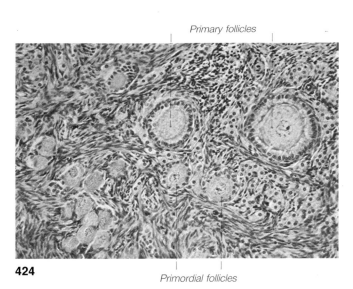

424

Primordial follicles

Membrana granulosa

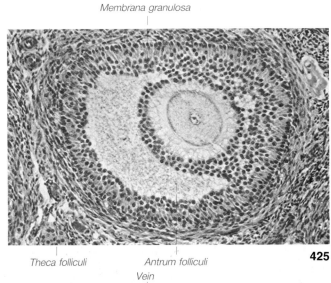

Theca folliculi *Antrum folliculi* **425**

Vein

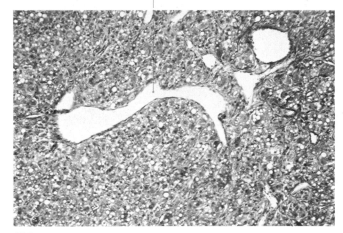

426

Lumen of vein

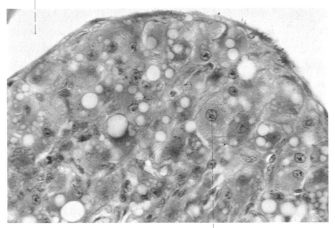

427 *Nucleus of granulosa lutein cell*

Fig. 424. Cortical zone of a human ovary showing several primordial and two primary follicles. The latter are characterized 1) by a higher and in later stages multilayered epithelium consisting of cuboidal or low columnar "granulosa" cells, 2) by a hyaline membrane (zona pellucida) interposed between the oocyte and the innermost layer of the granulosa cells and 3) by the larger size of the primary oocyte it contains. H & E staining. Magnification 150×.

Fig. 425. Secondary (antral) follicle with a crescent cavity (= antrum folliculi) and a developing cumulus oophorus. The cavity results from the progressive accumulation of fluid (liquor folliculi) among the granulosa cells of the multilayered follicular epithelium. The connective tissue immediately around the follicle has been transformed into cellular strands encircling the follicle, the theca folliculi. At a later stage, this layer will differentiate further into a theca interna and externa. H & E staining. Magnification 150×.

Fig. 426. Low-power view of the central part of a feline corpus luteum with several veins. The lipid droplets in the granulosa cells are dissolved out during routine histologic preparation and the cells thus appear highly vacuolated. Mallory-azan staining. Magnification 96×.

Fig. 427. A higher magnification from the center of the preceding micrograph better illustrates the large size of the granulosa lutein cells and their varying degree of vacuolization. Mallory-azan staining. Magnification 380×.

Female reproductive system – Uterine tube

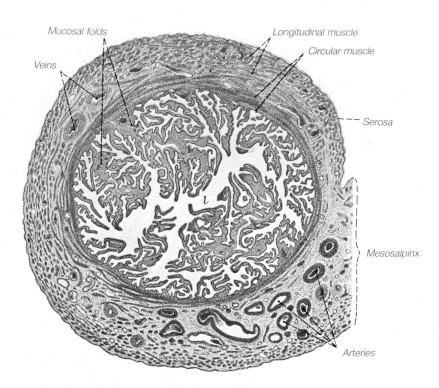

Fig. 428. Complete transverse section through a human uterine (fallopian) tube at the level of its ampulla (camera lucida drawing). Particularly characteristic are the delicate and highly-branched mucosal folds and the muscularis that is subdivided into rather indistinct layers. Only if the specimen is obtained intact and fixed with care will the outer serosal covering be preserved. See Table 15 for differentiation with other hollow organs. H & E staining. Magnification 22 ×.

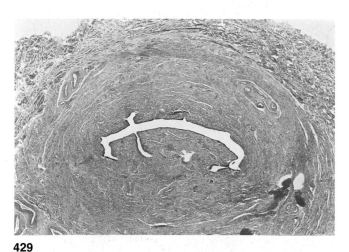

429

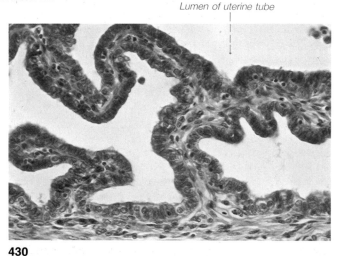

430

Fig. 429. Low-power light micrograph of complete cross-section through human fallopian tube at the level of its narrowest segment, the pars interstitialis. Notice absence of mucosal folds and a muscle coat consisting of more tightly gathered and predominantly circularly arranged smooth muscle cells as compared to the ampulla. H & E staining. Magnification 24 ×.

Fig. 430. Mucosal folds of a human uterine tube at higher magnification. The simple columnar epithelium is partly equipped with motile cilia (not seen in this figure, but in Figs. 80 and 92). The number of ciliated cells undergoing regular changes during the menstrual cycle. The subepithelial lamina propria consists of reticular connective tissue. H & E staining. Magnification 95 ×.

190

External uterine os   Cervical glands

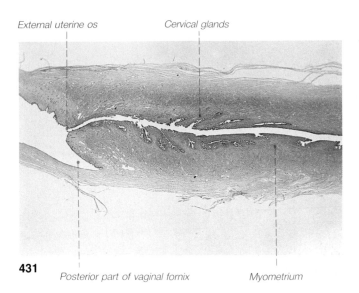

431   *Posterior part of vaginal fornix*   *Myometrium*

Endometrium with glands

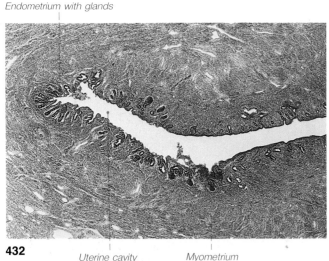

432   *Uterine cavity*   *Myometrium*
Lumen of cervical canal

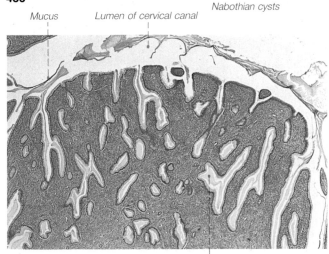

433   *Mucus*   *Lumen of cervical canal*   *Nabothian cysts*

434   *Glandular lumen filled with mucus*

Fig. 431. Longitudinal section through major parts (corpus and cervix) of a human virginal uterus (from 15-year-old girl) together with the upper end of the vagina (= fornix) which surrounds the vaginal portion of the cervix (=portio vaginalis cervicis). Notice slenderness of uterine cavity which opens via the cervical canal into the vagina at the external os. H&E staining. Magnification 5×.

Fig. 432. Higher magnification of the blind end of the uterine cavity from the same specimen as shown before (Fig. 431) reveals uterine mucosa (= endometrium) with early differentiation of simple tubular glands. H&E staining. Magnification 23×.

Fig. 433. Complete cross-section through vaginal portion of uterine cervix showing three Nabothian cysts. These rather large cavities (diameter up to several millimeters) develop if the ducts of several of the glands become occluded and the glands are then transformed into cysts by the accumulating secretory product. H&E staining. Magnification 5×.

Fig. 434. Higher magnification of the inner surface of the cervical canal from the preceding micrograph reveals numerous extensively branching tubular glands. They are lined by tall columnar epithelial cells (simple columnar epithelium) whose cytoplasm, like that of the surface epithelium, is filled with mucus. The latter is seen within the glandular lumina as well as covering the lining of the cervical canal. H&E staining. Magnification 23×.

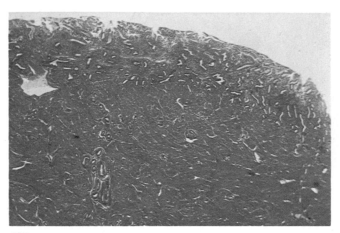

435

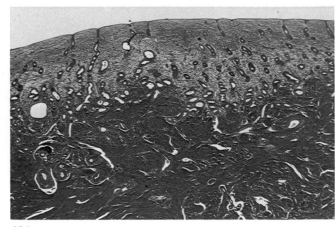

436

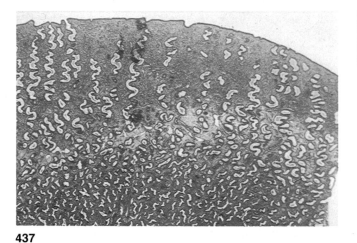

437

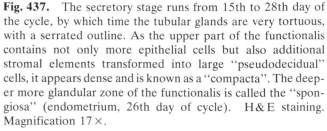

438

A set of micrographs to illustrate some of the characteristic appearances of the uterine mucosa (= endometrium) that occur regularly in each menstrual cycle.

Fig. 435. During the menstrual stage, ranging from the 1st to 4th day after the onset of menstruation, the "functionalis" is completely discarded. The surface epithelium is then restored by regeneration from the blind ends of the endometrial glands that always remain in the "basalis" (human uterus, 2nd day of menstruation). H & E staining. Magnification 17 ×.

Fig. 436. During the proliferative stage, from 5th to 14th day of the menstrual cycle, the upper portions (= functionalis) of the endometrium increase in thickness under the influence of ovarian estrogens. The basalis (approximately 1 mm thick) is only moderately involved in this growth period and is not discarded during later menstruation. During this phase the endometrial glands appear as straight tubules (human uterus, 12th day of cycle). H & E staining. Magnification 17 ×.

Fig. 437. The secretory stage runs from 15th to 28th day of the cycle, by which time the tubular glands are very tortuous, with a serrated outline. As the upper part of the functionalis contains not only more epithelial cells but also additional stromal elements transformed into large "pseudodecidual" cells, it appears dense and is known as a "compacta". The deeper more glandular zone of the functionalis is called the "spongiosa" (endometrium, 26th day of cycle). H & E staining. Magnification 17 ×.

Fig. 438. At higher magnification (detail from upper left corner of Fig. 437) the simple columnar epithelium is seen to be devoid of kinocilia. Note the intense cellularity of the compacta. H & E staining. Magnification 120 ×.

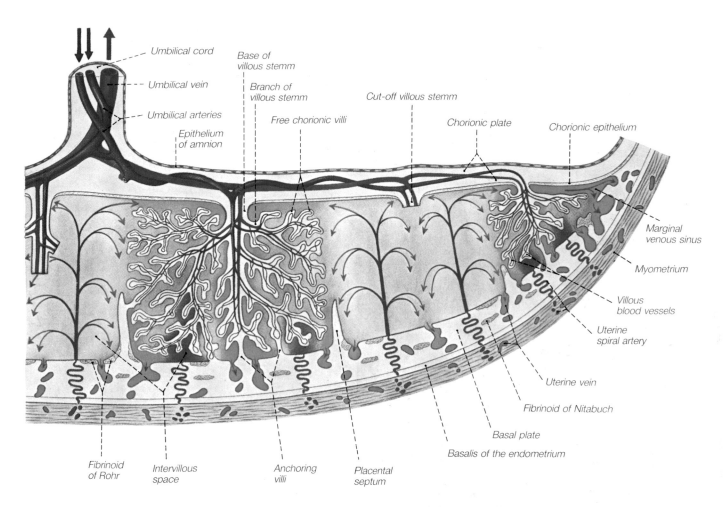

Umbilical cord

Umbilical vein

Umbilical arteries

Epithelium of amnion

Base of villous stemm

Branch of villous stemm

Free chorionic villi

Cut-off villous stemm

Chorionic plate

Chorionic epithelium

Marginal venous sinus

Myometrium

Villous blood vessels

Uterine spiral artery

Uterine vein

Fibrinoid of Nitabuch

Basal plate

Basalis of the endometrium

Fibrinoid of Rohr

Intervillous space

Anchoring villi

Placental septum

Fig. 439. Schematic presentation of the placental circulation (modified from von Heidegger and Starck). The blood enters intervillous spaces via the spiral arteries traversing the basal plate and then shoots upward onto the chorionic plate due to the high pressure it is under. Reflected at the chorionic plate it falls back and then circulates through the labyrinthic intervillous spaces, and is finally drained into the uterine veins. This is one of the rare examples of a truly "open" circulation in mammals, i.e., without a structured connecting link between the feeding and draining vessels of the system.

Female reproductive system – Placenta

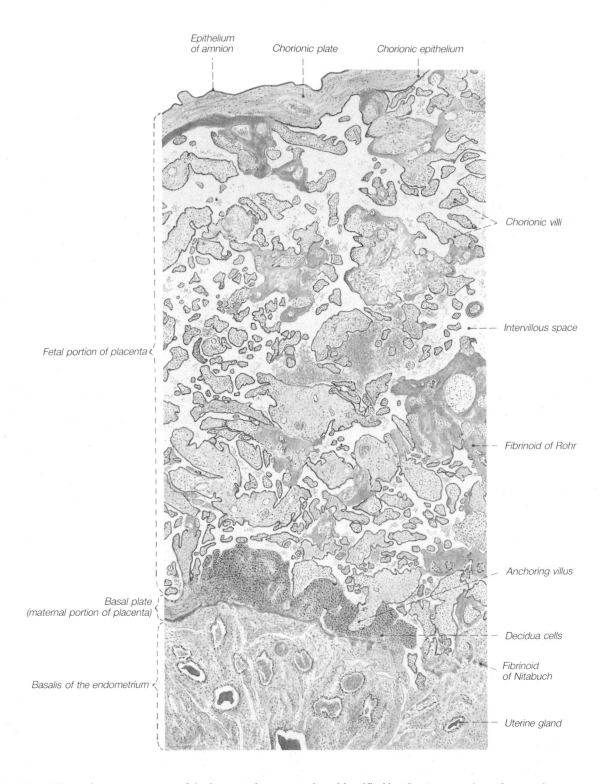

Epithelium
of amnion · Chorionic plate · Chorionic epithelium

Chorionic villi

Intervillous space

Fetal portion of placenta

Fibrinoid of Rohr

Anchoring villus

Basal plate
(maternal portion of placenta)

Decidua cells

Fibrinoid
of Nitabuch

Basalis of the endometrium

Uterine gland

Fig. 440. The various components of the human placenta are best identified in a low-power view of a complete cross-section of this complex organ. The fetal portion consists of 1) the chorionic plate, its two surfaces covered by the amniotic and chorionic epithelium and 2) the highly branching villous stems (= cotyledons) arising from the chorionic plate and partly attached to the opposing maternal surface by means of anchoring villi (see also Fig. 441). The maternal portion comprises 1) the basal plate, a derivative of the basal decidua, and 2) its septal projections (= placental septa) that form incomplete separations between individual cotyledons (camera lucida drawing). H & E staining. Magnification 27,5 ×.

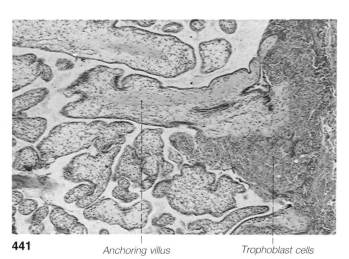

441   *Anchoring villus*   *Trophoblast cells*

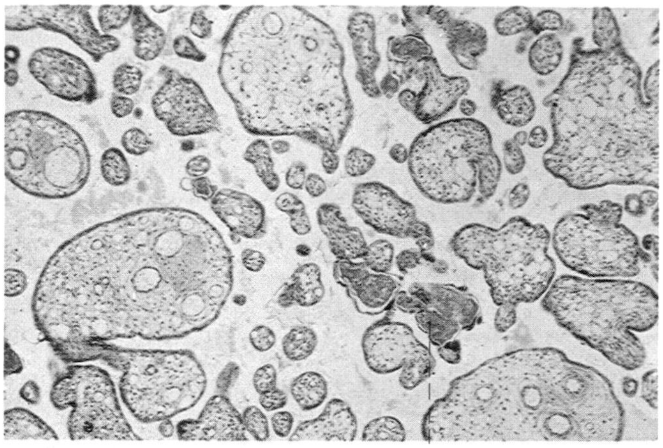

Fig. 441. Site of fusion between an anchoring villus and the basal plate (mature human placenta). The deeper staining orange strands coursing between the trophoblast cells are known as Nitabuch's fibrinoid (see also Fig. 440). Hematoxylin and chromotrop staining. Magnification 60×.

442   *Fibrinoid*

Fig. 442. Several cross-sectioned placental villi of different sizes from a mature human placenta. Note both the numerous vascular lumina seen within the connective tissue of the villi and the deposits of fibrinoid (stained orange) in the intervillous spaces. Hematoxylin and chromotrop staining. Magnification 60×.

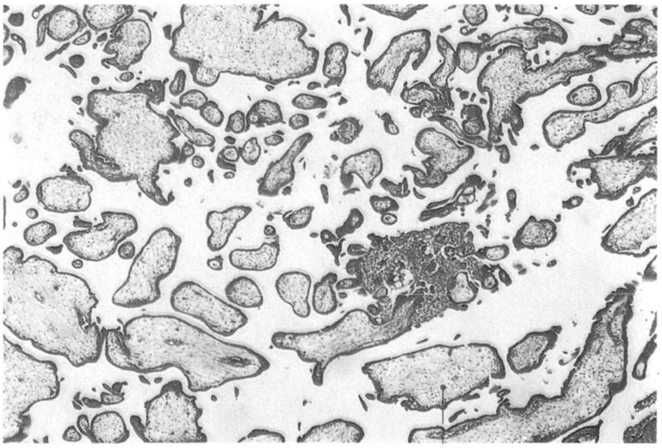

443   *Placental villus*

Fig. 443. Low-power view of an early human placenta in situ (about fourth month; fetus: 10 cm C.R. length). When compared to the fully matured organ (cf. Fig. 440) the absence of fibrinoid is a particularly striking feature recognizable at such low magnifications. H & E staining. Magnification 24×.

Fig. 444. Cross-sectioned villus from the same human placenta as shown before (Fig. 443). The surface is covered by a double-layered epithelium. The cells of the inner layer (= cytotrophoblast) give rise to those of the outer layer (= syncytiotrophoblast), the outer cells later fusing with each other. The large deeply stained cells in the connective tissue core are Hofbauer cells, closely related to histiqcytes. H & E staining. Magnification 240×.

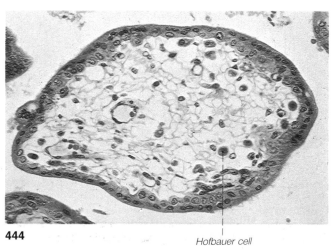

444   *Hofbauer cell*

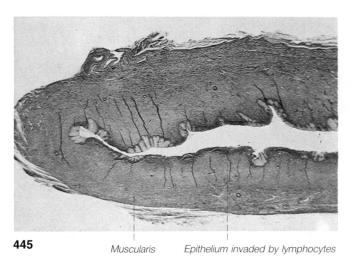

445   *Muscularis   Epithelium invaded by lymphocytes*

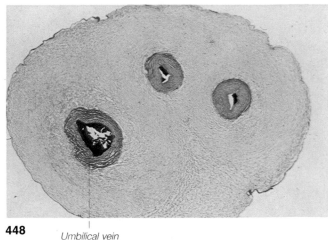

448   *Umbilical vein*

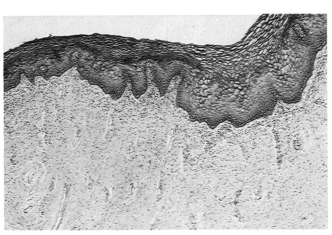

446

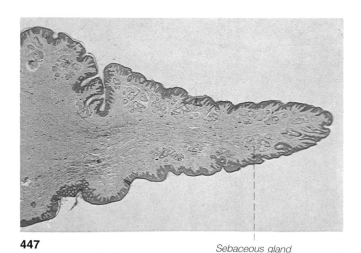

447   *Sebaceous gland*

Fig. 445. Transverse section through part of a human vagina to illustrate the composition of its wall. The stratified squamous noncornified epithelium (details shown in Fig. 81) is partly infiltrated by lymphoid aggregates. The thick connective tissue lamina propria never contains glands, but is rich in blood vessels, particularly venous plexuses. The muscularis consists of interlacing bundles of smooth muscle cells. For further identifying characteristics, see Figure 310. Mallory-azan staining. Magnification 7×.

Fig. 446. Vaginal epithelium is particularly rich in glycogen as can be shown by selective staining, e.g., deep red with Best's carmine as shown in this preparation. With desquamation of the epithelial cells, the glycogen is released into the vaginal lumen where it is metabolized to lactic acid by Döderlein's bacilli. Hematoxylin and Best's carmine staining. Magnification 60×.

Fig. 447. Cross-sectioned human minor labium which in contrast to the major labium never displays hairs or sweat glands, although it is rich in sebaceous glands. The stratified squamous epithelium is only slightly cornified and its basal cells are pigmented. H & E staining. Magnification 8×.

Fig. 448. Transverse section of a human umbilical cord obtained at delivery. The surface is covered by the simple amniotic epithelium, while embedded in its mucous connective tissue (= Wharton's jelly) are the two umbilical arteries and a single vein. As is usual after birth the three vessels are in a state of extreme contraction. No allantoic duct remnant is visible in this specimen. Mallory-azan staining. Magnification 10×.

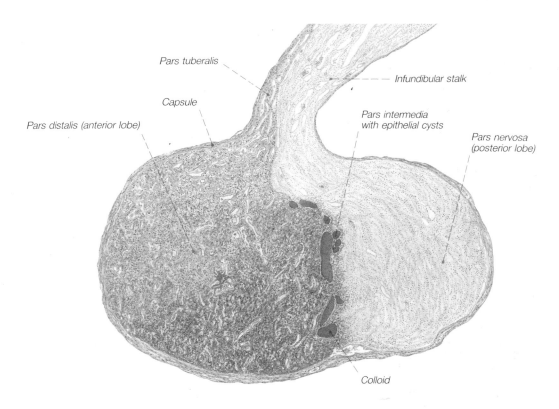

Pars tuberalis

Infundibular stalk

Capsule

Pars intermedia
with epithelial cysts

Pars distalis (anterior lobe)

Pars nervosa
(posterior lobe)

Colloid

Fig. 449. Low-power view of a complete midsagittal section through a human pituitary gland (= hypophysis) to demonstrate its different components. The adenohypophysis consists of the pars tuberalis (closely attached to the ventral aspect of the infundibular stalk), the pars distalis which represents the anterior lobe, and the pars intermedia (containing follicles filled with colloid). Missing from this preparation is the posterior part of the pars tubularis which covers the dorsal aspect of the infundibular stalk. Even at this very low magnification the non-random distribution of the various cell types of the anterior lobe is obvious because of the differences in staining reactions. The neurohypophysis consists of the infundibular stalk and the infundibular process (= pars nervosa). Camera lucida drawing. H & E staining. Magnification 10 ×.

Fig. 450. A slightly higher magnification again shows the uneven distribution of the cell types in the anterior lobe of the pituitary. Near the capsule (lower margin of the micrograph) chromophobe cells predominate, while centrally acidophils and groups of basophils prevail. To find examples of each cell type the low-power objective should be used to identify appropriate areas for more detailed examination. Preparations of the human pituitary, commonly obtained at autopsy, are often of poor quality because of post-mortem artifacts. Mallory-azan staining. Magnification 38 ×.

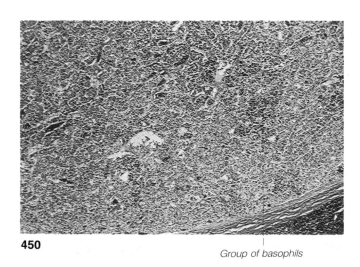

450

Group of basophils

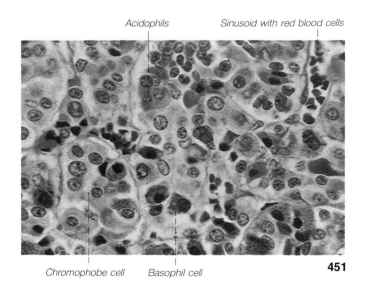

Acidophils   Sinusoid with red blood cells

Chromophobe cell   Basophil cell

451

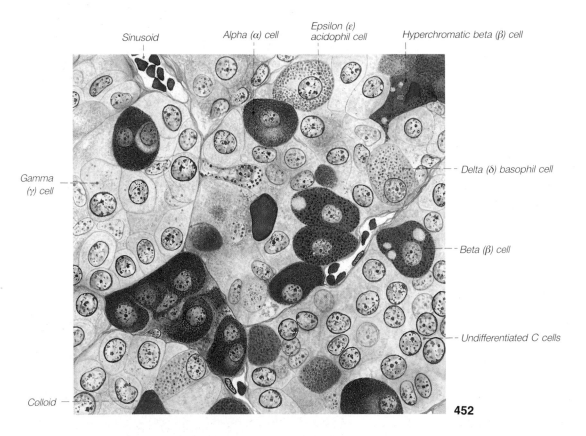

Sinusoid   Alpha (α) cell   Epsilon (ε) acidophil cell   Hyperchromatic beta (β) cell

Gamma (γ) cell

Delta (δ) basophil cell

Beta (β) cell

Undifferentiated C cells

Colloid

452

Figs. 451 and 452.   In a camera lucida drawing (Fig. 452) it is possible to illustrate all the cell types found in the anterior lobe of the human pituitary. Similar close groupings of these cells are seldom found in real histologic sections (Fig. 451), but most cell types can be identified by comparison with the drawing. In these particular specimens the usually red acidophils are rather orange in color. Staining: Mallory-azan (Fig. 451) and a special modification called "Kresazan" (Fig. 452). Magnifications 480 × (Fig. 451) and 980 × (Fig. 452).

198

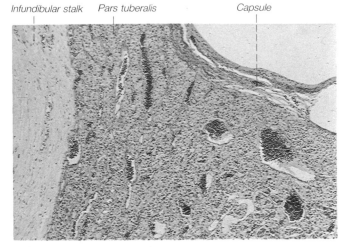

Infundibular stalk *Pars tuberalis* *Capsule*

453

Fig. 453. The pars tuberalis and adjacent infundibular stalk from a mid-sagittal section of human pituitary. In contrast to the anterior lobe, the pars tuberalis consists of uniform cells arranged in cords with numerous intervening blood vessels. The vessels have wide lumina and are part of the hypophyseal portal system. Mallory-azan staining. Magnification 60 ×.

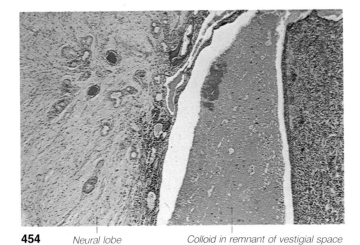

454 *Neural lobe*   *Colloid in remnant of vestigial space*

Fig. 454. Low-power view of the pars intermedia (human pituitary), predominantly occupied by a large cyst whose colloid contents are separated from its epithelial wall by a broad cleft caused by the removal of water during the embedding procedure. To the right of the cyst are the adjoining parts of the anterior lobe, while to the left remnants of the intermediate lobe (small cellular strands and cysts) blend with the pars nervosa (= neural part of the gland). Mallory-azan staining. Magnification 38 ×.

Colloid in epithelial cyst

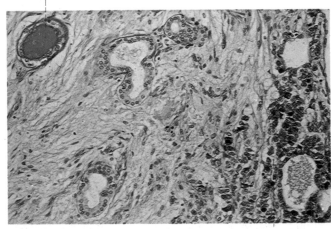

455   *Basophils of pars intermedia*

Fig. 455. A higher magnification of part of the middle third of the preceding micrograph illustrates more clearly the epithelial cysts, one of which contains colloid, and highly basophilic cells of the pars intermedia merging with the pars nervosa. The cellular and fiber organization of the neural lobe are only seen with special staining procedures. Mallory-azan staining. Magnification 150 ×.

199

Endocrine glands – Epiphysis cerebri

Sand granules (Acervulus)

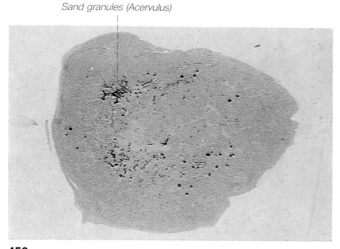

456

Fig. 456. Low-power view of a complete sagittal section through the human pineal body (= epiphysis cerebri). Since well preserved specimens are difficult to obtain, the pineal is often not demonstrated in histology courses. The gland may be confused with the parathyroid, especially when the specimen is not thoroughly studied at low-power. Differentiating features are 1) the considerably larger size of the pineal (cf. Fig. 462), 2) the poorer staining of the pineal due to its high nerve fiber content and faintly staining cells and 3) the more prominent connective tissue septa that clearly separate the pineal cells into lobules. Sand granules (acervulus), although unique to the pineal, are focal in disposition and thus may be missed unless the section is first studied at low magnification. H & E staining. Magnification 10 ×.

457

Figs. 457 and 458. At higher magnification, conventionally stained specimens of pineal show that the cells are arranged in groups, but they do not allow to distinguish between the specific pinealocytes and glial cells. The cells of the pineal are not closely apposed to each other and the gland thus lacks the clearly epithelial structure seen in the parathyroid (cf. Fig. 463). In the middle of Figure 458 are two cross-sectioned capillaries each containing an erythrocyte. H & E staining. Magnifications 150 × and 380 ×, respectively.

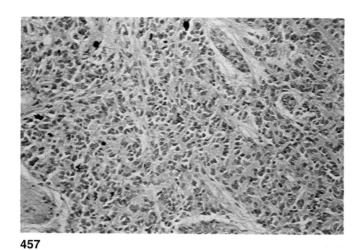

458

Blood capillary

Fig. 459. Because of its lobular organization and the close resemblance of its follicles to alveolar secretory units, the thyroid is occasionally confused with a lactating mammary gland (for differentiation, see Figs. 418–421 and Table 14). In most specimens, the follicles are seen in varying stages of activity from empty to filled with colloid (human thyroid). Mallory-azan staining. Magnification 38 ×.

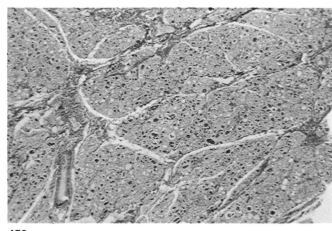

459

Collapsed follicle

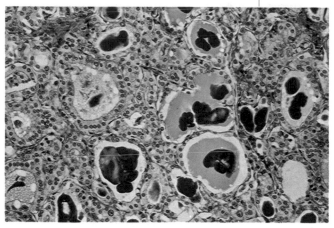

460

Fig. 460. Higher magnification of the same specimen (Fig. 459) shows the variable staining reactions of the colloid, even within the same follicle. These reflect the varying water content of the colloid; with increasing age, the water content is reduced and the colloid stains redder with azocarmine. The separation of colloid from the follicular epithelium is an artifact due to dehydration of the colloid during tissue preparation. Mallory-azan staining. Magnification 150 ×.

Fig. 461. Several small empty follicles (human thyroid) between which can be seen a few of the parafollicular cells that produce the hormone calcitonin. Parafollicular cells can easily be simulated by tangential sections through small follicles and are thus readily confused with them. Mallory-azan staining. Magnification 480 ×.

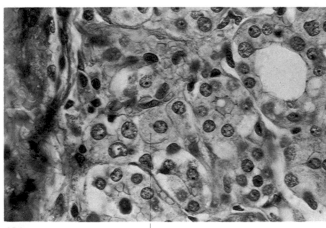

461

Parafollicular cell

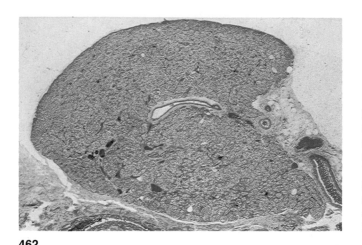

462

Fig. 462. Sections of the human parathyroid usually display adherent thyroid tissue. When, as in this complete midsagittal section, the parathyroid is shown in isolation it can be confused with the pineal gland. The parathyroid can be distinguished by 1) its smaller size, 2) its lesser amount of more delicate interstitial connective tissue and 3) its closely attached, darker staining and obviously epithelial parenchymal cells (cf. Figs. 456–458). Hematoxylin and phloxine staining. Magnification 38×.

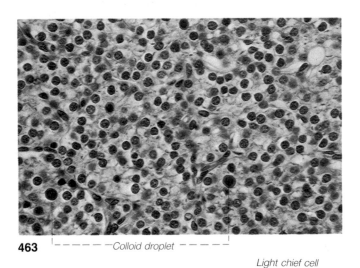

463 |‒ ‒ ‒ ‒ ‒Colloid droplet ‒ ‒ ‒ ‒ ‒|

Fig. 463. The epithelial nature of the parenchymal cells of the human parathyroid is seen better at higher magnification. The individual cells differ in the intensity of their staining reactions. The two particularly acidophilic globules indicated in the lower third of the micrograph are colloid droplets found occasionally in this gland. Mallory-azan staining. Magnification 380×.

Light chief cell

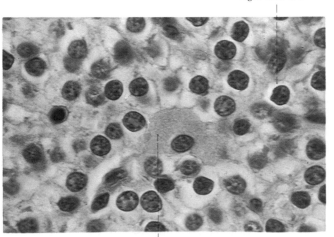

464   Oxyphil cell

Fig. 464. The majority of the epithelial cells of the human parathyroid are chief cells, designated "light" or "dark" by the staining reaction of their cytoplasm. "Dark" chief cells are thought to represent the active secretory stage. In the center of the micrograph is one of the rare oxyphil cells of the parathyroid. This particular example shows less cytoplasmic acidophilia than usual and lacks the characteristic pyknotic nucleus. Mallory-azan staining. Magnification 960×.

202

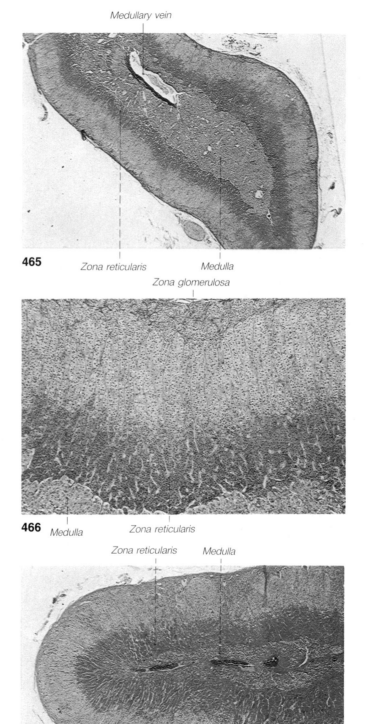

Fig. 465. When viewed with the naked eye or at very low power as here, cross-sections of the adrenals show a characteristic layered organization. In this specimen there appear to be three layers; 1) an outer faintly staining layer, 2) a middle darker stained zone and 3) an inner paler area. The last corresponds to the adrenal medulla, while the first two are both cortical (see also Fig. 466). The large veins equipped with thick muscular walls are characteristic of the medulla. Mallory-azan staining. Magnification 15×.

Fig. 466. Only at higher magnification can the three different zones of the adrenal cortex be identified. Because of the arrangement of their cells they are known as 1) zona glomerulosa (cells gathered into ovoid packets), 2) zona fasciculata (cells aligned in parallel cords) and 3) zona reticularis (cells forming a network). The zona reticularis stains particularly well and may thus be mistaken for the medulla (human adrenal). Mallory-azan staining. Magnification 48×.

Fig. 467. If a fresh adrenal is immersed in a fixative containing potassium bichromate, the medullary cells become brown and are therefore known as chromaffin cells (pig adrenal). The reaction is due to the oxidation of the epinephrine and norepinephrine stored in these cells in granular form. In this specimen the zona reticularis is clearly defined by its darker staining. Nuclear fast red staining after potassium bichromate fixation. Magnification 24×.

203

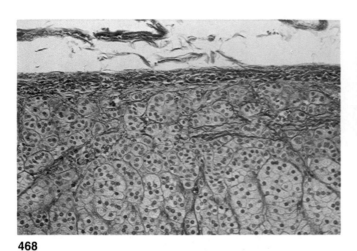

468

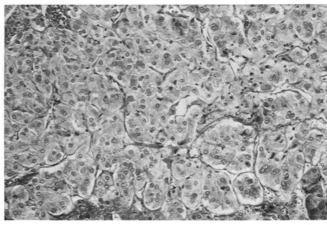

471

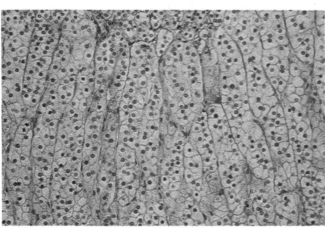

469

Details of the three cortical zones and the medulla from the same human adrenal.
All figures: Mallory-azan staining. Magnification 150×.

Fig. 468. Subjacent to the thin connective tissue capsule is the narrow zona glomerulosa comprising small ovoid groups of cuboidal cells enveloped by a fine network of reticulin fibers extending from the capsule throughout the cortex. Those zona glomerulosa cells closest to the capsule are thought to be poorly differentiated elements forming a "cortical blastema".

Fig. 469. The cells of the zona fasciculata are arranged in parallel cords. They contain numerous lipid droplets, but since these are dissolved out during processing the cells have a vacuolated appearance (= spongiocytes). See also Figure 55.

Fig. 470. The deeper staining cells of the zona reticularis are arranged in interconnecting cords forming a network (reticulum) containing numerous blood vessels. Along the lower edge of the micrograph are seen the outermost layers of the medulla.

Fig. 471. The medullary cells arise from the sympathetic primordia and thus correspond to a paraganglion. As is usual in ordinary preparations, their intracytoplasmic granules are not seen. They become obvious when furnished with a brown tinge by oxidation as with potassium bichromate (see Fig. 467) and are therefore known as chromaffin or pheochrome cells (pheos, Gr. = brown).

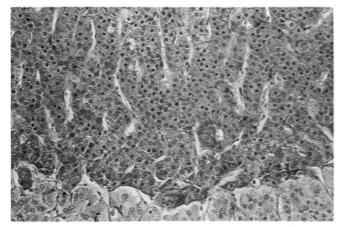

470

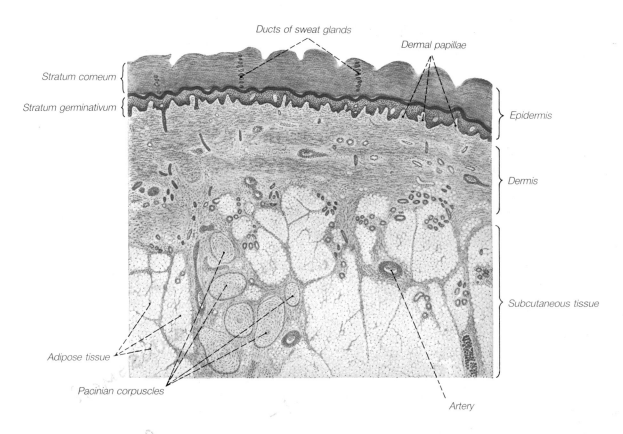

Ducts of sweat glands

Dermal papillae

Stratum corneum

Stratum germinativum

Epidermis

Dermis

Subcutaneous tissue

Adipose tissue

Pacinian corpuscles

Artery

Fig. 472. The lamination of the human skin is particularly well seen in heavily cornified regions such as palms and soles. There are two main layers, the epidermis and the underlying dermis (= corium). At this magnification the epidermis can be roughly separated into a superficial cornified layer (= stratum corneum), an intermediate deeper staining band (= stratum granulosum plus stratum lucidum) and a deep cellular layer (= stratum germinativum). The dermis is composed of connective tissue, the superficial (= papillary) layer of which serves as a mechanical device for the firm attachment of the epidermis. The deeper (= reticular) layer of the dermis contains not only coarser collagen fiber bundles, but also the majority of the glands and blood vessels of the skin (camera lucida drawing). H & E staining. Magnification 18 ×.

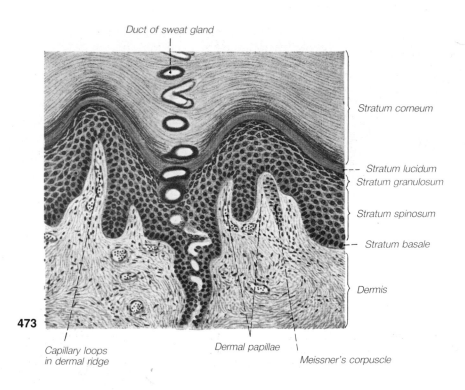

Duct of sweat gland

Stratum corneum

Stratum lucidum
Stratum granulosum

Stratum spinosum

Stratum basale

Dermis

473

Capillary loops
in dermal ridge

Dermal papillae

Meissner's corpuscle

Fig. 473. The detailed lamination of the epidermis is seen at higher magnification; 1) the stratum basale or germinativum comprising columnar cells arranged in a single layer and the overlying 2) stratum spinosum together form the stratum malpighii. Above this is 3) the stratum granulosum which stands out because of its deeply staining keratohyalin granules. Next is the highly re-fractile 4) stratum lucidum and most superficially 5) the stratum corneum. In the stratum corneum the keratohyalin granules have merged with the tonofilaments to form a filament-matrix complex, while the cell membranes have thickened and the nuclei and other organelles have vanished completely (camera lucida drawing). H & E staining. Magnification 17 ×.

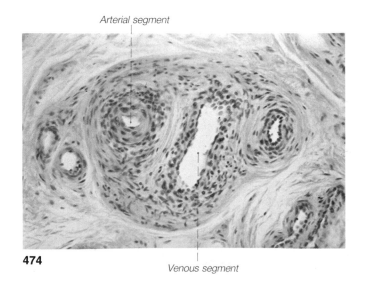

Arterial segment

474

Venous segment

Fig. 474. Transverse section through a glomus (= organ of Hoyer-Grosser) in the reticular layer of the dermis of a human finger tip. This specialized component of the microvascular bed consists of a coiled arteriovenous anastomosis with a particular rich innervation, all enclosed within a fibrous capsule. H & E staining. Magnification 150 ×.

206

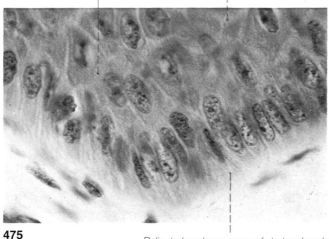

"Intercellular bridges" in the stratum spinosum

475   *Delicate basal processes of stratum basale*

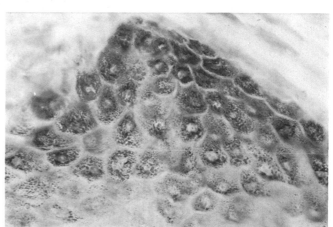

476   *Delicate cytoplasmic spines in the stratum spinosum*

Fig. 475. The columnar epithelial cells of the stratum basale extend slender cytoplasmic processes into the underlying connective tissue to achieve a firm attachment to it (cf. Fig. 63 b). Above the basal cells, the "intercellular bridges" between the prickle cells of the stratum spinosum are faintly visible (epidermis of human finger tip). H & E staining. Magnification 960 ×.

Fig. 476. During tissue processing the cells of the stratum spinosum shrink. At the same time they remain attached to each other by desmosomes (cf. Fig. 63 a), which results in their apparent studding by many spiny processes. The cells are thus often called prickle cells (human condyloma accuminatum). Iron hematoxylin staining. Magnification 960 ×.

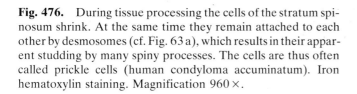
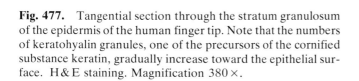

477

Fig. 477. Tangential section through the stratum granulosum of the epidermis of the human finger tip. Note that the numbers of keratohyalin granules, one of the precursors of the cornified substance keratin, gradually increase toward the epithelial surface. H & E staining. Magnification 380 ×.

Fig. 478. Non-human material is commonly used to demonstrate intracellular tonofibrils (epithelial matrix of the hoof of bovine fetus). Each tonofibril consists of subunits, the tonofilaments (see Fig. 48 b). The tonofibrils serve as a cytoskeleton of individual cells and, because of their arrangements along the lines of major mechanical stress, collectively strengthen the epithelium. Iron hematoxylin staining. Magnification 380 ×.

Epithelial nuclei

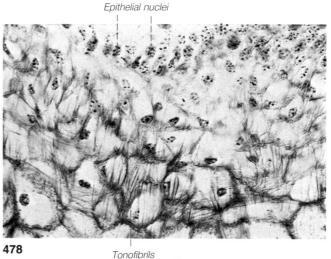

478   *Tonofibrils*

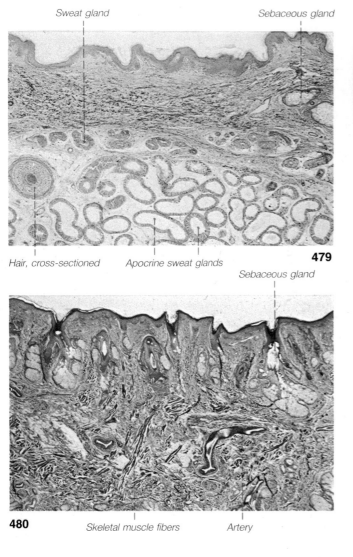

Sweat gland · Sebaceous gland

Hair, cross-sectioned · Apocrine sweat glands · **479**

Sebaceous gland

480 Skeletal muscle fibers · Artery

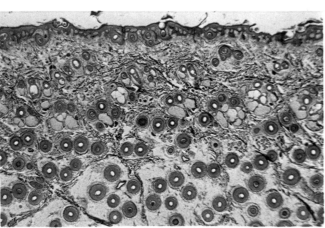

481

Tunica dartos

482 · Apocrine sweat glands

Certain areas of the integument such as the axillary region and the skin of the palms or soles, the scalp, the scrotum and the labia can be identified because of characteristic morphologic features.

Fig. 479. The axillary skin has a thin, poorly cornified epithelium together with hairs and sebaceous and sweat glands. The most characteristic feature is the large number of apocrine sweat glands, identified by their wide lumina and the varying height of their secretory cells (details shown in Figs. 105, 488, 489). Iron hematoxylin and benzopurpurin staining (slightly faded). Magnification 38×.

Fig. 480. Skin from a human nostril. Typical for this area are the numerous sebaceous glands that are not associated with hairs. For detailed identifying characteristics see Table 11. Mallory-azan staining. Magnification 20×.

Fig. 481. The skin of the human scalp is easily identified by its large complement of closely spaced hairs (see also Fig. 483). Since the hairs lie oblique to the surface, a perpendicular section will cut through them at different levels so that their cross-sections vary greatly in appearance. Mallory-azan staining. Magnification 17×.

Fig. 482. Skin of the human scrotum with the characteristic layer of smooth muscle (tunica dartos) that clearly distinguishes this cutaneous area from all others. In addition, apocrine and merocrine sweat glands together with sebaceous glands occur in varying numbers and occasional hairs may be found. Iron hematoxylin staining. Magnification 38×.

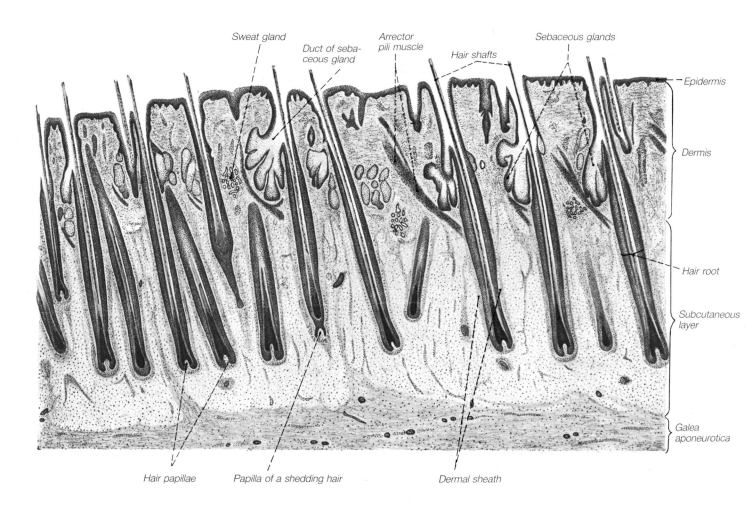

Sweat gland

Duct of seba-
ceous gland

Arrector
pili muscle

Hair shafts

Sebaceous glands

Epidermis

Dermis

Hair root

Subcutaneous
layer

Galea
aponeurotica

Hair papillae

Papilla of a shedding hair

Dermal sheath

Fig. 483. Longitudinal sections through the hairs of a human scalp show their free ends (= shafts) projecting above the surface while their roots are embedded in deep invaginations (= hair follicles) each consisting of an epithelial and a connective tissue sheath (camera lucida drawing). H & E staining. Magnification 40×.

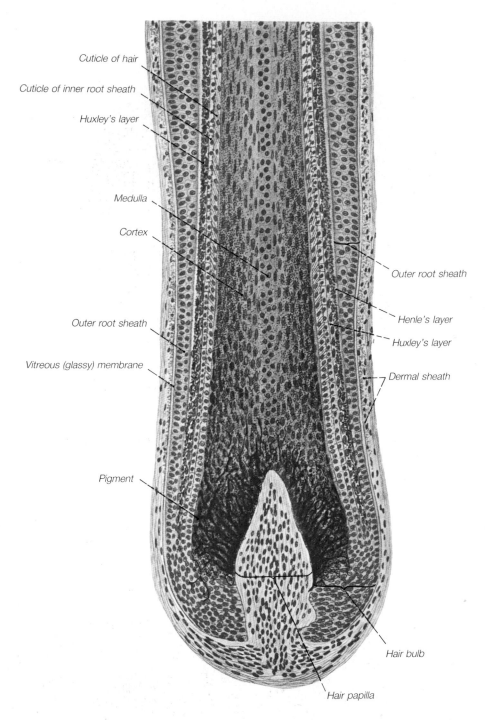

Cuticle of hair

Cuticle of inner root sheath

Huxley's layer

Medulla

Cortex

Outer root sheath

Outer root sheath

Vitreous (glassy) membrane

Henle's layer

Huxley's layer

Dermal sheath

Pigment

Hair bulb

Hair papilla

Fig. 484. A higher magnification shows the rather complex layering of the epithelial part of the hair follicle, divided into an inner and an outer root sheath. The inner root sheath consists of 1) the cuticle of the root sheath which interdigitates with the hair cuticle firmly anchoring the hair root within its sheath and 2) Huxley's layer of one or two rows of elongated cells attached to 3) Henle's layer, a single row of flattened cells. The outer or external root sheath is continuous with the stratum germinativum of the epidermis and its outermost cylindrical cells are covered by the vitreous (or hyaline) membrane that forms the inner layer of the connective tissue sheath of the hair follicle (camera lucida drawing). H & E staining. Magnification 200 ×.

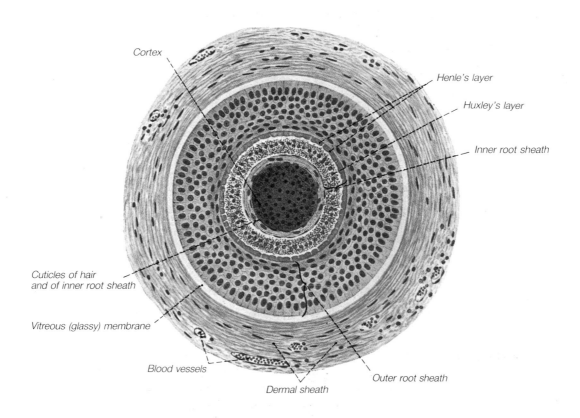

Fig. 485. Transverse section through the hair root showing its various sheaths (camera lucida drawing). Compare with Figure 484. H & E staining. Magnification 300×.

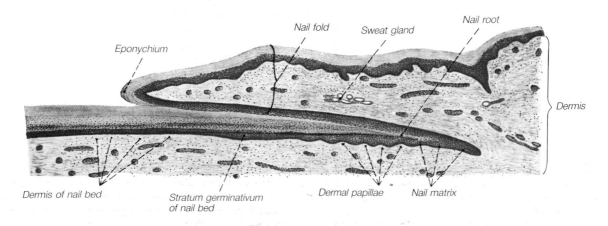

Fig. 486. Longitudinal section of the proximal parts of a newborn's nail (camera lucida drawing). H & E staining. Magnification 30×.

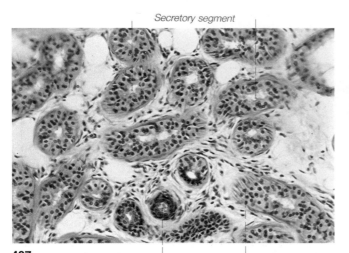

Secretory segment

487
Cellular apices with secretion product   Origin of excretory duct   Myoepithelial cells

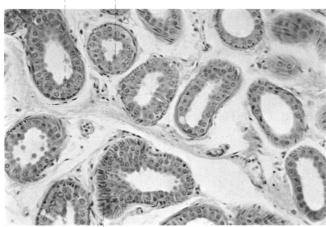

Cytoplasmic hoods formed by the apocrine secretion mechanism

488   Myoepithelial cells

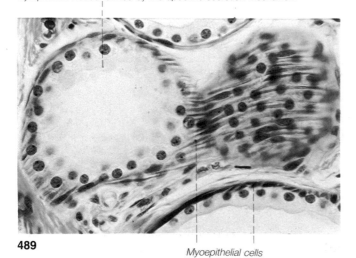

489   Myoepithelial cells

490

Fig. 487. The merocrine sweat glands, located mostly at the border between the dermis and the subcutaneous tissue, are simple tubular glands whose distal parts are tightly coiled (see Fig. 99). Compared to the secretory portions, the long excretory ducts have narrower lumina lined by deeper staining cells with closer spaced nuclei. Note the myoepithelial cells that appear as discrete "stripes" at the bases of tangentially sectioned secretory tubules. H & E staining. Magnification 150×.

Fig. 488. Apocrine sweat glands are branched alveolar glands found only in certain areas of the skin (human axillary skin). They are characterized by the wide lumina of their secretory portions and by the variation in glandular epithelial height, the latter assumed to be the structural equivalent of the different stages of an apocrine secretion mechanism (cf. Figs. 105, 479). H & E staining. Magnification 150×.

Fig. 489. The spindle-shaped contractile myoepithelial cells are particularly well demonstrated in tangential sections of the secretory alveoli of apocrine sweat glands, although the cells are not unique to these glands (human ceruminous glands). Mallory-azan staining. Magnification 380×.

Fig. 490. Holocrine sebaceous glands are also branched alveolar in type, but their lumina are usually packed with masses of epithelial cells gradually transforming into the secretory product, the sebum. Mallory-azan staining. Magnification 60×.

The integument – Mammary gland

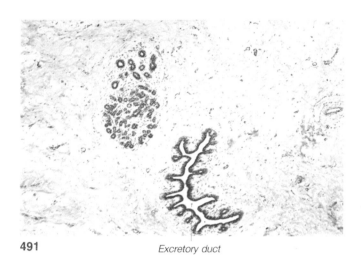

491   *Excretory duct*

Excretory duct

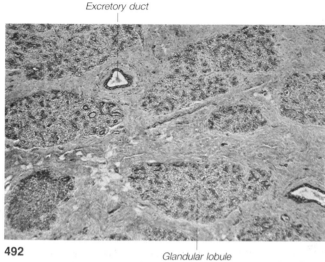

492   *Glandular lobule*

Fig. 491. Part of a resting mammary gland showing a larger excretory duct and a cluster of secretory alveoli surrounded by a thin fibrous capsule. H&E staining. Magnification 38×.

Fig. 492. The proliferating mammary gland of a pregnant woman. Under the influence of various hormones during pregnancy the epithelial tubules of the resting gland beginn to increase in size and number, compressing the regressing connective tissue into thin strands that persist as interlobular septa carrying the larger blood vessels and excretory ducts. H&E staining. Magnification 38×.

Adipose tissue   *Excretory duct*

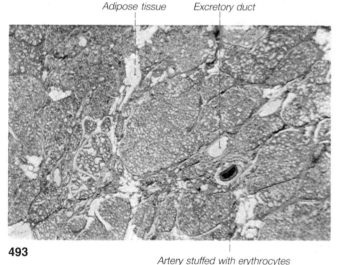

493

Artery stuffed with erythrocytes

Fig. 493. The mammary gland is fully developed only in lactation. It consists of 10–15 separate tubulo-alveolar glands, whose secretory parts vary considerably in size due to their different stages of activity. Profiles of the larger excretory ducts are regularly found within the interlobular connective tissue septa. For other characteristics, see Figures 418–421 and Table 14. Mallory-azan staining. Magnification 34×.

Fig. 494. Because routine embedding procedures involve lipid solvents, the cells of the active secretory alveoli show numerous vacuoles instead of fat droplets. Although the alveolar contents occasionally resemble thyroid colloid, the mammary alveoli can always be distinguished from thyroid follicles by their very irregular outlines. Mallory-azan staining. Magnification 150×.

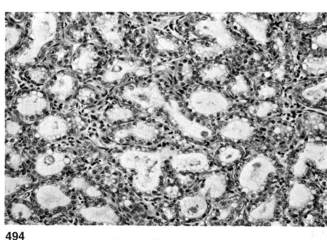

494

213

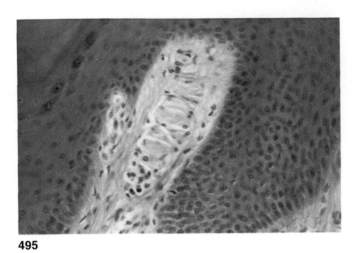

495

Fig. 495. Longitudinal section of a tactile corpuscle of Meissner from human finger tip. These corpuscles are located in the dermal papillae, especially in hairless skin. They consist of a stack of elongated club-shaped connective tissue cells between which an afferent axon persues its spiral course. H & E staining. Magnification 240 ×.

Axon

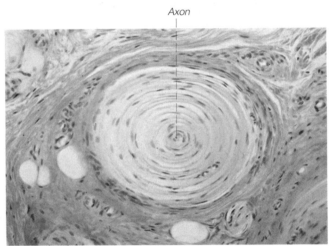

496

Fig. 496. Transverse section through a Pacinian corpuscle (human finger tip), another receptor for mechanical stimuli. These are found predominantly in the deeper layers of the subcutaneous tissue. They are composed of a single central axon surrounded by a large number of concentric cellular lamellae separated from one another by interstices filled with a clear fluid. Iron hematoxylin and benzopurpurin staining. Magnification 150 ×.

Connective tissue capsule

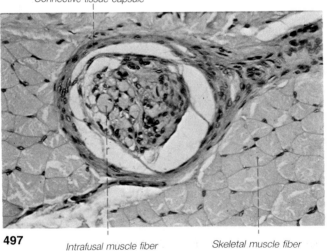

497

Intrafusal muscle fiber   Skeletal muscle fiber

Fig. 497. Cross-section of a muscle spindle from a human lumbrical muscle. Like the two preceding examples, these receptors possess a prominent connective tissue capsule in this case enclosing a number of so-called "intrafusal" fibers. The fibers are arranged parallel to the ordinary muscle fibers, but are smaller with a non-contractile midportion and a special innervation. Hematoxylin staining. Magnification 240 ×.

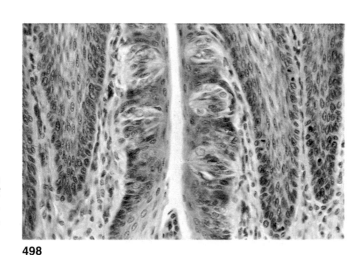

498

Fig. 498. Several taste buds situated in the epithelium lining a trench between foliate papillae (rabbit tongue). Because of their poor stainability, these sensory organs show at low magnifications as cone-shaped translucencies within the darker epithelium. Iron hematoxylin staining. Magnification 290×.

Nucleus of a neuroepithelial (taste) cell

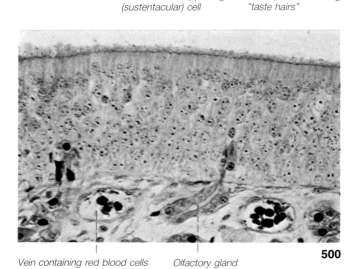

499

Fig. 499. At higher magnification two cell types can be distinguished within taste buds by their different nuclear sizes (rabbit foliate papilla). The supporting (sustentacular) cell contains a large rounded nucleus and its apical portion does not regularly reach the taste pore. The taste cell has a more elongated deeper staining nucleus and always reaches into the taste pore with an apical process (= "taste hair"), a bunch of slender microvilli. Because of the thickness of this section, the "taste hairs" appear as a homogeneous blackening along the bottom of the taste pore. Iron hematoxylin staining. Magnification 960×.

Nucleus of a supporting (sustentacular) cell   *Taste pore containing "taste hairs"*

Fig. 500. The pseudostratified columnar epithelium of the olfactory mucosa (canine olfactory region) differs from respiratory epithelium in being thicker and free of goblet cells. As in the human, this epithelium consists of sustentacular and olfactory cells, the latter being bipolar ganglion cells although difficult to identify as such in routine preparations. In this specimen details of the apical processes of the olfactory cells, such as the olfactory vesicles and motile cilia, are obscured by the mucus covering the epithelial surface and by the thickness of the section. Iron hematoxylin and benzo light Bordeaux. Magnification 380×.

Vein containing red blood cells   *Olfactory gland*

500

215

Organs of the special senses – Eye

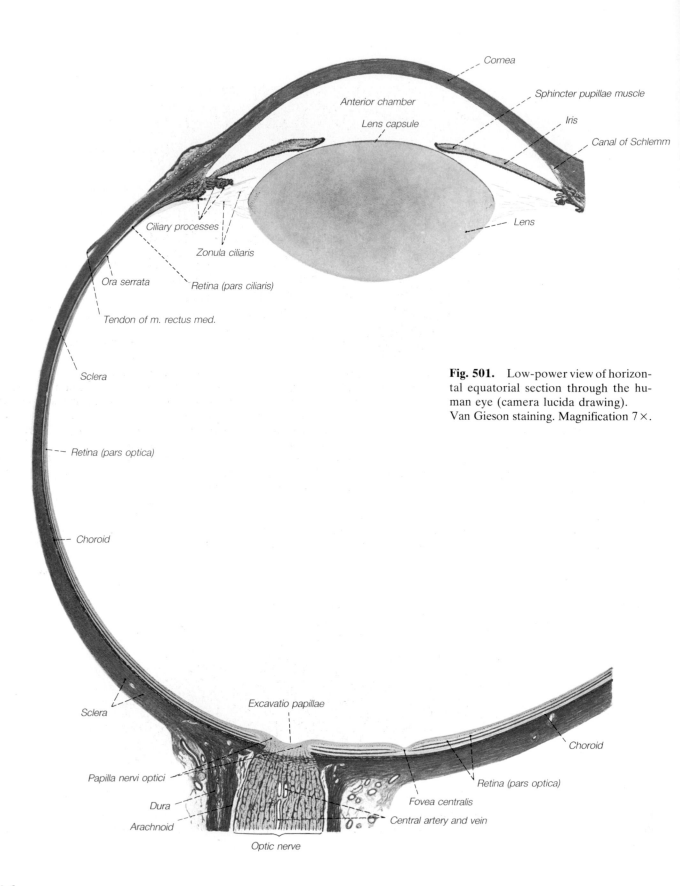

Cornea

Anterior chamber

Sphincter pupillae muscle

Lens capsule

Iris

Canal of Schlemm

Ciliary processes

Lens

Zonula ciliaris

Ora serrata

Retina (pars ciliaris)

Tendon of m. rectus med.

Fig. 501. Low-power view of horizontal equatorial section through the human eye (camera lucida drawing). Van Gieson staining. Magnification 7×.

Sclera

Retina (pars optica)

Choroid

Sclera

Excavatio papillae

Choroid

Papilla nervi optici

Retina (pars optica)

Dura

Fovea centralis

Arachnoid

Central artery and vein

Optic nerve

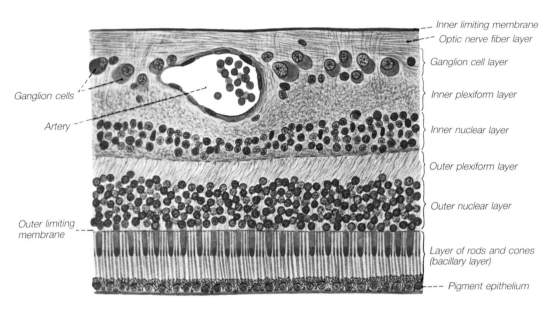

Inner limiting membrane
Optic nerve fiber layer
Ganglion cell layer
Inner plexiform layer
Ganglion cells
Inner nuclear layer
Artery
Outer plexiform layer
Outer nuclear layer
Outer limiting membrane
Layer of rods and cones (bacillary layer)
Pigment epithelium

Fig. 502. The apparently complex stratification of the light-sensitive part of the retina is due to an orderly sequence of three separate, but interconnected, neuron types. In order of conduction of impulses, the first neurons are those in the outermost layer, viz. the photoreceptor or rod and cone cells. Moving inward there follow the two layers of nerve cells and their processes that are the second and third neurons of the optic tract. The nuclei and the processes of all three neurons occur in separate well-defined levels of the retina producing the stratification. The outer and inner nuclear layers and the ganglion cell layer, respectively, contain the cell bodies and nuclei of 1) the rod and cone cells, 2) the bipolar neurons and 3) the multipolar ganglion cells of the optic nerve. The plexiform layers contain the processes of the neurons in the adjoining layers. In the outer plexiform layer the axons of the rod and cone cells (first neuron) make synaptical contacts with the dendrites of the bipolar (second) neurons, while the inner plexiform layer contains synapses formed between the bipolar neuronal axons and the ganglion cell (third neuron) dendrites. The innermost retinal layer consists of the axons of the ganglion cells converging towards the papilla, where they form the optic nerve. The retina also contains specific glial cells (= supporting Müller cells), although these are not seen in routine preparations. The inner and outer limiting membranes are formed, respectively, by the expanded ends of slender processes of Müller cells and by an elaborate system of intercellular adhesive devices established between the Müller cells and the outer segments of the photoreceptors (camera lucida drawing). H & E staining. Magnification 400 ×.

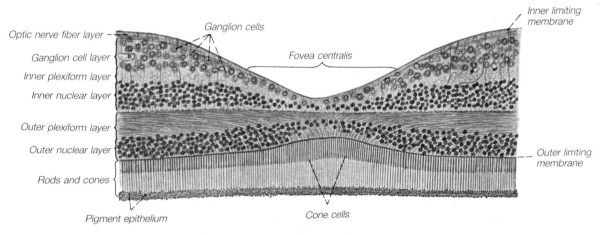

Inner limiting membrane
Optic nerve fiber layer
Ganglion cells
Fovea centralis
Ganglion cell layer
Inner plexiform layer
Inner nuclear layer
Outer plexiform layer
Outer nuclear layer
Outer limiting membrane
Rods and cones
Pigment epithelium
Cone cells

Fig. 503. Section through the central fovea in the macula lutea (= region of maximum visual acuity). The inner layers of the retina deviate at this site thus allowing light more direct access to the photoreceptors that in this area consist only of cones (camera lucida drawing). H & E staining. Magnification 175 ×.

Pigment epithelium   Ganglion cell layer

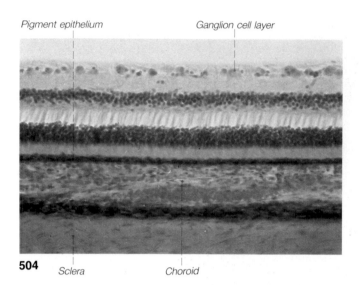

504

Sclera   Choroid

Fig. 504. Human retina in situ with adjoining pigment epithelium, choroid and inner parts of sclera. Use Figures 502–503 to identify the various layers. H&E staining. Magnification 240×.

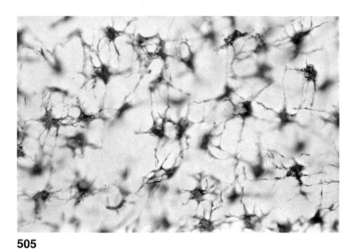

505

Fig. 505. Tangential section through a human cornea. The tissue has been impregnated with gold chloride to illustrate the highly branched fibroblasts (= keratocytes) interspersed in the substantia propria. Magnification 240× (specimen courtesy of Prof. H. J. Clemens, Munich).

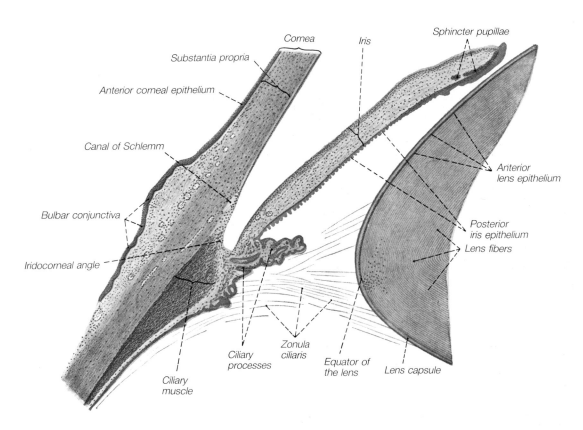

Fig. 506. Part of a horizontal equatorial section through the anterior part of the eyeball (cf. Fig. 501) showing the ciliary body, anterior and posterior chambers, iris, lens, and corneal rim (camera lucida drawing). H & E staining. Magnification 35 ×.

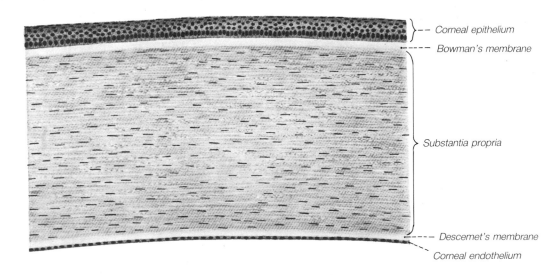

Fig. 507. The cornea normally contains no blood vessels and its stroma (= substantia propria) consists mostly of connective tissue fibers with modified fibroblasts (= keratocytes) of which only the nuclei are visible. The branching cell bodies can be demonstrated by special methods, such as gold impregnation (see Fig. 505). The isolated cornea is often used for the simultaneous demonstration of a stratified and a simple squamous epithelium (camera lucida drawing). H & E staining. Magnification 80 ×.

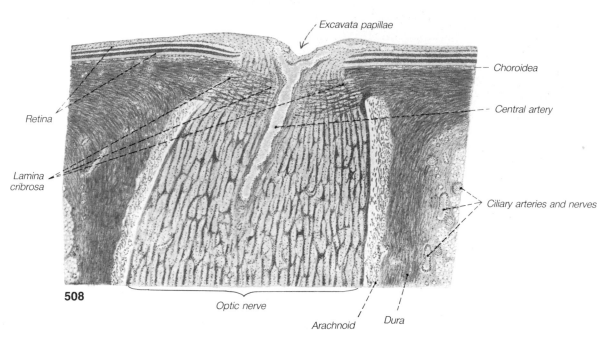

Excavata papillae

Choroidea

Central artery

Retina

Lamina cribrosa

Ciliary arteries and nerves

508

Optic nerve

Arachnoid   Dura

Fig. 508. Camera lucida drawing of a longitudinal section of human optic nerve head with optic disk (= papilla nervi optici) and its central indentation (= excavatio papillae). Van Gieson staining. Magnification 20×.

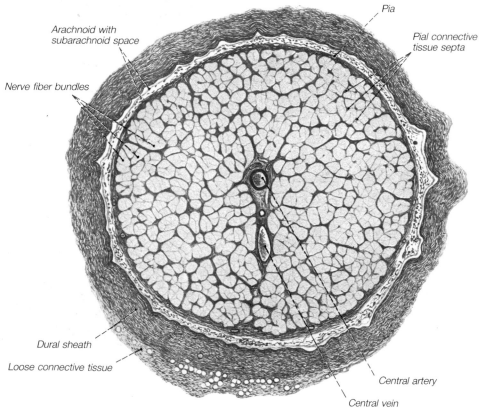

Pia

Arachnoid with subarachnoid space

Pial connective tissue septa

Nerve fiber bundles

Dural sheath

Loose connective tissue

Central artery

Central vein

Fig. 509. Cross-section of the optic nerve which as a part of the brain is ensheathed by the three meninges and a subarachnoid space. The presence of a central artery and vein should not be used as an absolute criterion for the identification of the optic nerve, as these vessels only enter the nerve about half an inch behind the eye (camera lucida drawing). Van Gieson staining. Magnification 22×.

220

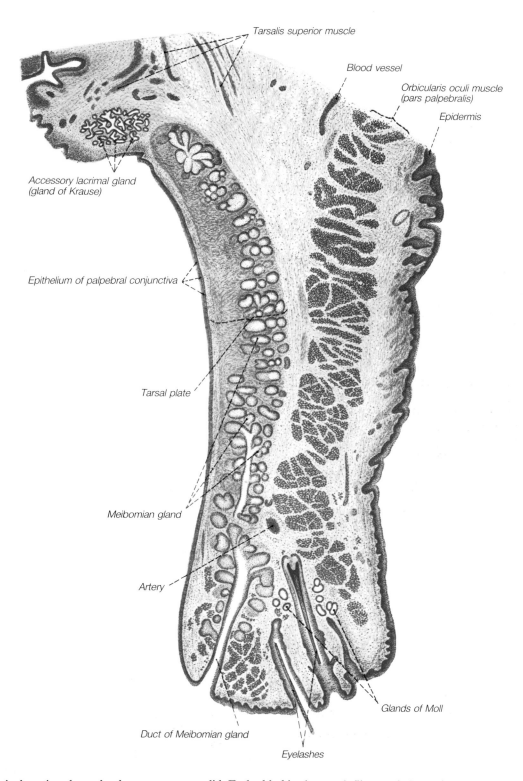

Tarsalis superior muscle

Blood vessel

Orbicularis oculi muscle
(pars palpebralis)

Epidermis

Accessory lacrimal gland
(gland of Krause)

Epithelium of palpebral conjunctiva

Tarsal plate

Meibomian gland

Artery

Glands of Moll

Duct of Meibomian gland

Eyelashes

Fig. 510. Vertical section through a human upper eyelid. Embedded in the tough fibrous skeleton (= tarsal plate) are sebaceous (= Meibomian) glands arranged in a single row with their long axes perpendicular to the lid margin. Apocrine sweat glands (of Moll) are only found close to the lashes. Attached to the upper border of the tarsal plate is the involuntary superior tarsal muscle of Müller, whose tone keeps the lid open (camera lucida drawing). For further identifying characteristics see Table 11. H & E staining. Magnification 17 ×.

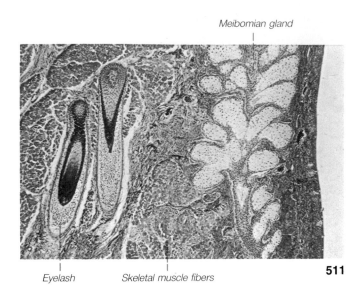

Meibomian gland

Eyelash   *Skeletal muscle fibers*   **511**

Fig. 511. Detail of human eyelid (vertical section) near the lid margin. At the right is seen the low palpebral conjunctival epithelium followed by a profile of a Meibomian gland, the cross-sectioned fibers of the orbicularis oculi muscle and parts of two eyelashes. Mallory-azan staining. Magnification 38×.

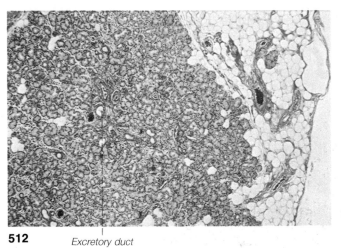

512   *Excretory duct*

Fig. 512. The lumina of the secretory parts of the human lacrimal gland are clearly visible at low magnification, unlike all other serous glands, e.g., parotid and pancreas. The lacrimal gland is a tubulo-alveolar gland, further characterized by a simple duct system in which only intra- and interlobular excretory ducts are found. For further identifying characteristics see Figs. 307–309 and Table 12. Mallory-azan staining. Magnification 38×.

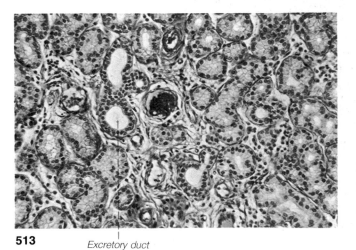

513   *Excretory duct*

Fig. 513. The secretory cells of the alveoli have spherical nuclei similar to those of the serous alveoli of the parotid gland. The connective tissue interstices contain numerous lymphocytes and groups of plasma cells (see also Fig. 122). Mallory-azan staining. Magnification 150×.

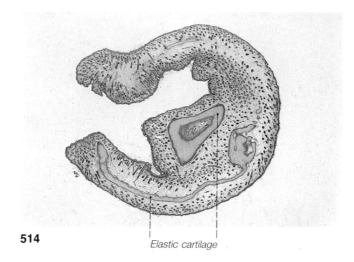

Fig. 514. Plane section through the pinna (= auricle) of a human fetus (approx. fifth month). It consists of a plate of elastic cartilage covered by a thin skin with primordia of hairs and glands. H & E staining. Magnification 18 ×.

514

Elastic cartilage

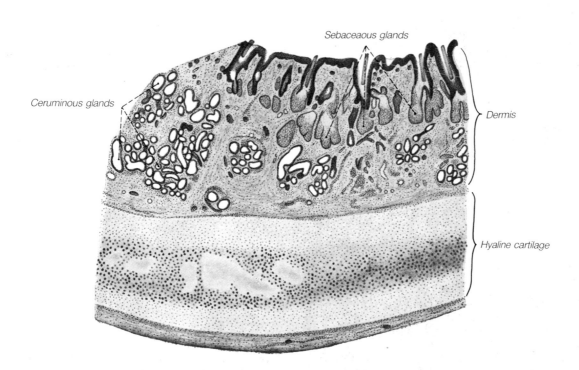

Sebaceaous glands

Ceruminous glands

Dermis

Hyaline cartilage

Fig. 515. Part of a cross-section through the cartilaginous portion of a human external auditory meatus (camera lucida drawing). It is lined by skin which shows not only hairs associated with sebaceous glands, but numerous large alveolar ceruminous glands that are a variety of apocrine sweat glands. Details of ceruminous glands are shown in Figs. 104 and 489. H & E staining. Magnification 16 ×.

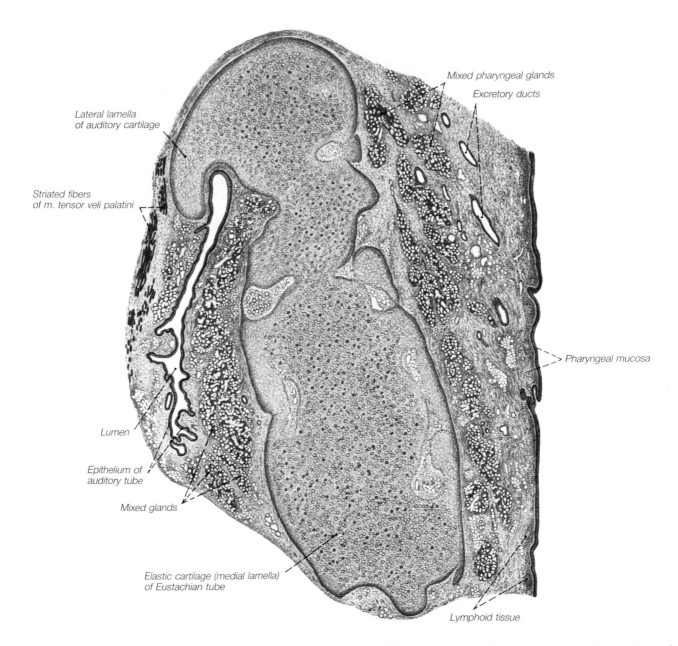

Mixed pharyngeal glands

Excretory ducts

*Lateral lamella
of auditory cartilage*

*Striated fibers
of m. tensor veli palatini*

Pharyngeal mucosa

Lumen

*Epithelium of
auditory tube*

Mixed glands

*Elastic cartilage (medial lamella)
of Eustachian tube*

Lymphoid tissue

Fig. 516. Cross-section through the cartilaginous part of the auditory (= Eustachian) tube. The mucosa consists of a pseudostratified columnar ciliated epithelium in which there are goblet cells and the lamina propria contains lymphoid aggregates that increase in number towards the pharyngeal opening. The mucosal glands are seromucous in nature and the cartilage predominantly elastic (camera lucida drawing). H & E staining. Magnification 13 ×.

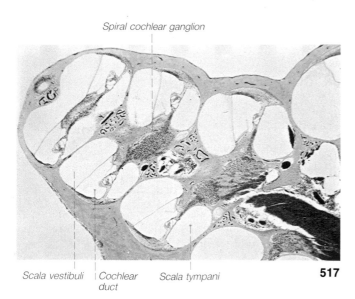

Spiral cochlear ganglion

Scala vestibuli | Cochlear duct | Scala tympani   **517**

518   Basilar membrane   Scala tympani   Spiral cochlear ganglion
Outer tunnel   Outer hair cells   Tectorial membrane

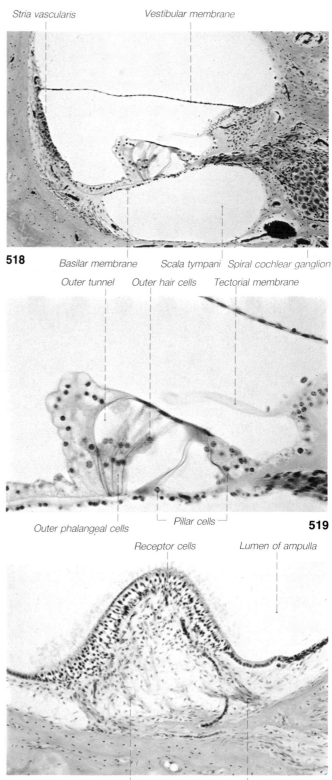

Stria vascularis   Vestibular membrane

Outer phalangeal cells   Pillar cells   **519**

Receptor cells   Lumen of ampulla

520   Myelinated nerve fibers

Fig. 517. Axial section through the cochlear canal (guinea pig) which in man makes about two and a half turns round a central column (= modiolus) that contains regularly spaced profiles of the cross-sectioned spiral ganglion (bipolar nerve cells) and the auditory nerve. Level with each ganglion profile a bony shelf (= osseous spiral lamina) projects from the modiolus. Mallory-azan staining. Magnification 24 ×.

Fig. 518. Cross-section through one turn of the bony cochlear canal (guinea pig) showing three fluid-filled cavities, the middle one (= cochlear duct) representing the cochlear extension of the membranous labyrinth and filled with endolymph. Two perilymphatic spaces run in parallel, a lower scala tympani and an upper scala vestibuli. The upper wall of the cochlear duct is formed by the delicate vestibular membrane (of Reissner), the lower wall mainly by the membranous spiral lamina and the outer wall by the richly vascular stria vascularis that is thought to produce the endolymph. Mallory-azan staining. Magnification 96 ×.

Fig. 519. Higher magnification of the auditory receptor (= organ of Corti) that consists of sensory (hair) cells and various supporting cells (pillar, phalangeal, border, Hensen and Claudius cells). Clearly visible are the three cavities that extend the length of the cochlea, from right to left the inner tunnel, the space of Nuel and the outer tunnel. In addition, inner and outer pillar cells (more eosinophilic), outer phalangeal and outer hair cells and the cells of Hensen and Claudius can all be identified. The epithelium covering the spiral limbus is continuous with both the tectorial membrane and the epithelium lining the internal spiral sulcus. Mallory-azan staining. Magnification 240 ×.

Fig. 520. Crista ampullaris of a semicircular canal from a guinea pig. The cupula has been lost in this section, but the myelinated fibers of the vestibular nerve are easily visible in the connective tissue core of the crista. Mallory-azan staining. Magnification 150 ×. (Specimen for Figs. 517–520 courtesy of Prof. L. Thorn, Munich).

Dorsal root

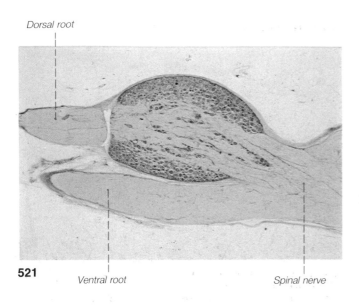

521

Ventral root

Spinal nerve

Fig. 521. Longitudinal section through a canine spinal ganglion. The ganglion is bisected by the longitudinally sectioned myelinated nerve fibers of the dorsal root that join those of the ventral root to form the spinal nerve. Cresyl violet staining. Magnification 21×.

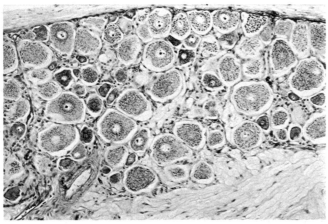

522

Fig. 522. The bodies of the sensory neurons are situated mostly at the periphery of the ganglia, their axons forming the dorsal or afferent root of the spinal nerve. Most of the cells are rather large and more or less spherical pseudounipolar nerve cells. The smaller, darker staining neurons are richer in lipids and are thought to be responsible for the conduction of protopathic sensory impulses (canine spinal ganglion). Cresyl violet staining. Magnification 120×.

Axon hillock

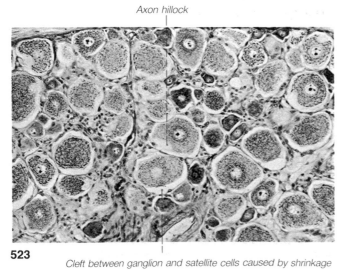

523

Cleft between ganglion and satellite cells caused by shrinkage

Fig. 523. The pseudounipolar ganglion cells show prominent axon hillocks and a homogeneous distribution of their finely granular Nissl substance. Each of the neurons is invested by a layer of flattened glial cells akin to Schwann cells, but often these "satellite" cells become separated from the neuronal body by shrinkage artifact. Cresyl violet staining. Magnification 150×.

226

Small group of ganglion cells

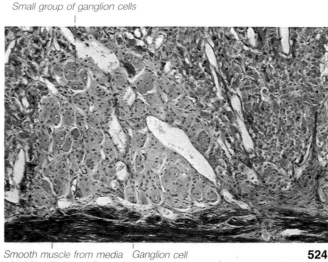

Smooth muscle from media   Ganglion cell   **524**
of thick walled medullary vein

Fig. 524. Autonomic ganglion from human adrenal medulla. Minute aggregates of multipolar autonomic neurons are particularly frequent at this site because as a derivative of the sympathetic primordium, the medulla is one of the chromaffin paraganglia. The neurons are easily identified by the large size of their cell bodies and nuclei with prominent nucleoli. Mallory-azan staining. Magnification 95×.

Bundle of nerve fibers of the myenteric plexus   Smooth muscle

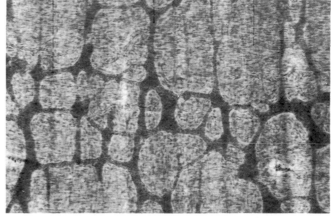

525

Fig. 525. Flat preparation of the myenteric plexus (of Auerbach) that is situated between the outer and inner layers of the intestinal muscularis externa. Non-myelinated nerve bundles of different sizes form this network at the intersections of which small groups of autonomic (parasympathetic) ganglion cells are found. Supravital staining with methylene blue. Magnification 95×.

Bundle of autonomic nerve fibers with two small ganglion cells   Ganglion cell

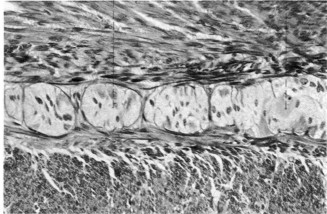

526
Smooth muscle, cross-sectioned

Fig. 526. Cross-section of the myenteric plexus from human colon. A few small ganglion cells are located between the nonmyelinated autonomic nerves. Mallory-azan staining. Magnification 240×.

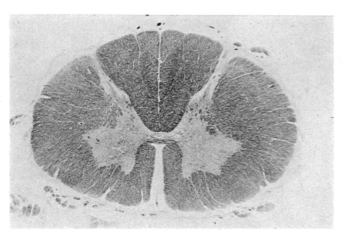

527

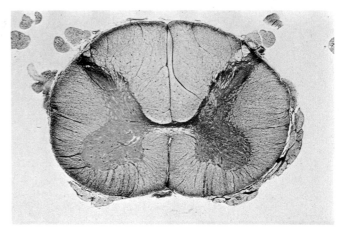

530

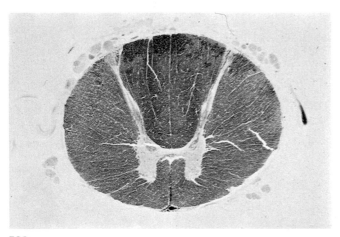

528

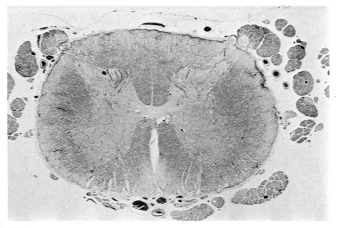

529

Figs. 527–529. Transverse section through cervical, thoracic and lumbar segments of the human spinal cord, all stained similarly for myelin and all shown at the same magnification (6×). Since the myelinated nerve fibers have been blackened, the white matter appears darker than the gray matter. Note the variation in the size and shape of the gray matter and the presence of a lateral gray column in the thoracic segment. See Figures 531 and 533 for nomenclature. Staining: Weigert's method for myelin.

Fig. 530. Cross-section of a cervical segment from a human spinal cord treated with a silver impregnation technique to illustrate the neurofibrils.

In specimens stained with the Nissl method for nerve cells, the tissue as a whole appears almost colorless when viewed with the naked eye. In such cases the student should use the lowest-power objective to find one of the anterior gray columns because these are particularly rich in neuron cell bodies. Silver impregnation after Schultze-Stöhr. Magnification 6×.

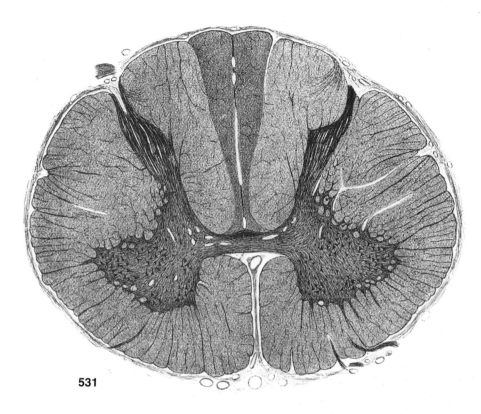

531

Fig. 531. Cross-section through the cervical enlargement of a human spinal cord (camera lucida drawing). The white matter on each side is subdivided into 1) the posterior funiculus lying between the posterior median septum and the posterior gray column, 2) the lateral funiculus between the posterior and anterior gray columns and roots and 3) the anterior funiculus located between the anterior gray column and the anterior median fissure. Staining: Carmine. Magnification 8 ×.

Fig. 532. Transverse section through a human medulla at the level of the upper third of the olive. The section has been stained for myelinated nerves so that the tightly folded olivary nucleus appears almost uncolored, while the cross-sectioned pyramidal tracts are obvious as massive fiber bundles close to the midline. Staining: Weigert's method for myelin. Magnification 6 ×.

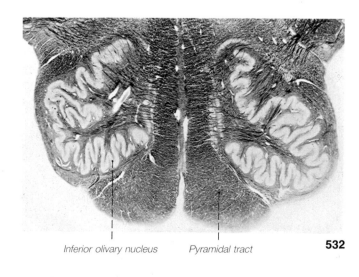

Inferior olivary nucleus   *Pyramidal tract*   **532**

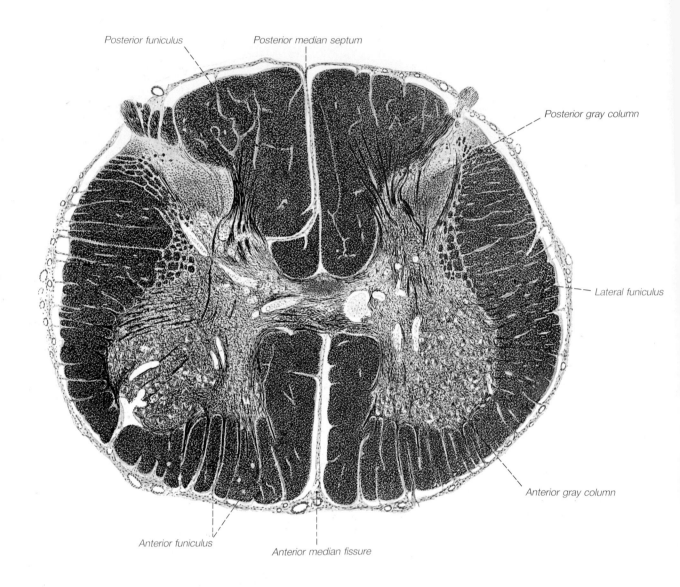

Posterior funiculus

Posterior median septum

Posterior gray column

Lateral funiculus

Anterior gray column

Anterior funiculus

Anterior median fissure

Fig. 533. Cross-section through the lumbar enlargement of a human spinal cord. Staining: Carmine combined with Weigert's method for myelin. Magnification 11×.

White matter

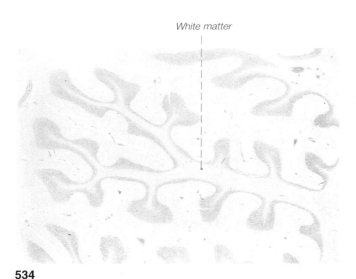

534

White matter

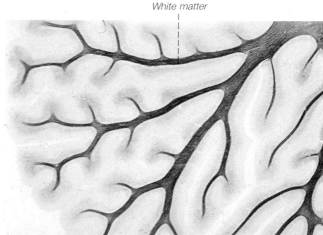

535

Figs. 534–536. Sagittal sections through the cortex of a human cerebellar vermis shown at the same magnification (7 ×), but with different stains.

The highly cellular granular layer stands out particularly clearly as a greyish-blue band with the Nissl method (Fig. 534) that stains only nerve cells and glial nuclei, while myelin stain (Fig. 535) outlines the centrally located white matter and its ramifications. Only by combining a stain for cells with one for myelin (Fig. 536) are the layering of the cerebellar cortex and its demarcation from the central white matter clearly illustrated. The cortex is approximately 1 mm thick and consists of 1) an outer molecular layer (stained a yellow orange) rather poor in cells, 2) an intermediate layer of Purkinje cells and 3) an inner granular layer (reddish brown) rich in nerve cells and bordering on the white matter.

Staining (from top to bottom): Nissl method, Weigert's method for myelin, carmine combined with the Weigert method.

White matter

536 *Molecular layer*   *Granular layer*

┌ *Purkinje cell dendrites* ┐

Fig. 537. A higher magnification illustrates the thick fanned-out Purkinje cell dendrites that reach up to the cerebellar surface. The Purkinje cell axon arises at the lower pole of the perikaryon and crosses the granular layer to terminate in one of the cerebellar nuclei. Staining: Silver impregnation (Bodian). Magnification 240 ×.

537

231

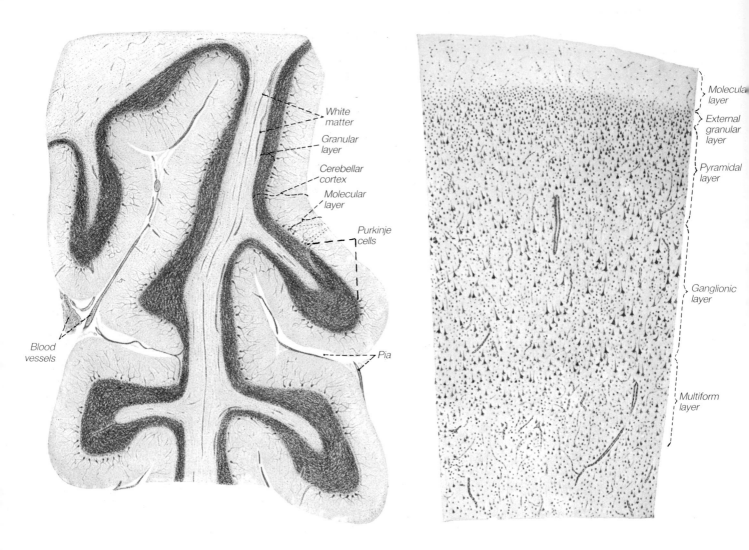

Fig. 538. Low-power view to demonstrate the lamination of the cerebellar cortex with a simple cell stain (camera lucida drawing). Carmine staining. Magnification 20×.

Fig. 539. Slightly schematized drawing of the cellular layers of the human motor cortex. Because of the prominence of the pyramidal layers and the near absence of granular layers, this is an "agranular" cortex. See also Figure 541. Carmine staining. Magnification 20×.

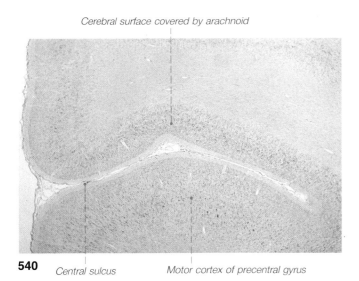

540 *Central sulcus*   *Motor cortex of precentral gyrus*

Cerebral surface covered by arachnoid

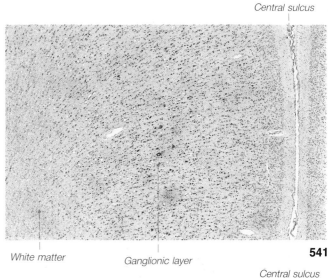

Central sulcus

White matter   *Ganglionic layer*   **541**

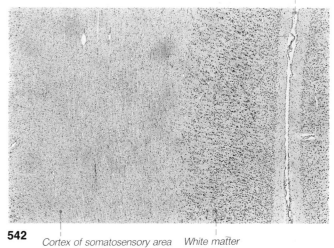

Central sulcus

542 *Cortex of somatosensory area*   *White matter*

Fig. 540. Central sulcus of baboon cerebral hemisphere with pre- and postcentral gyrus. The cortex (in this case neopallium or isocortex) consists uniformly of six superimposed nerve cell layers which vary in thickness and distinctness. In addition, the demarcation between gray matter (cortex) and white matter is less prominent in the precentral gyrus. Nissl staining (with Toluidine blue). Magnification 8.5×.

Fig. 541. Higher magnification of the precentral gyrus (somatomotor area) of the preceding micrograph shows two pyramidal layers the inner of which (= ganglionic layer) contains particularly large cells known as giant pyramidal cells of Betz (see also Fig. 543). Due to the poorly developed, granular layers the motor cortex belongs to the "agranular" type of isocortex. Nissl staining. Magnification 24×.

Fig. 542. Significantly reduced cortical thickness (to less than 50% of that seen in the motor cortex) and less distinct pyramidal layers together with a clear-cut demarcation between cortex and underlying white matter are characteristic features of the postcentral gyrus (somatosensory area). Nissl staining. Magnification 24×.

Fig. 543. Giant pyramidal cell of Betz from ganglionic layer of the human motor cortex. Cresyl violet staining. Magnification 240×.

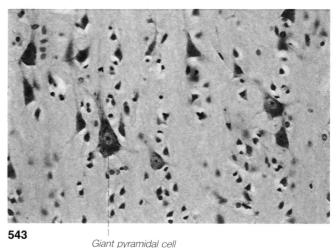

543   *Giant pyramidal cell*

233

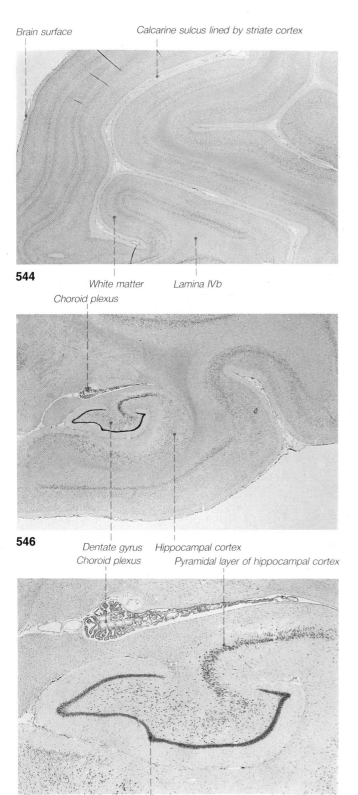

Brain surface | Calcarine sulcus lined by striate cortex

544

White matter | Lamina IVb

Choroid plexus

546

Dentate gyrus | Hippocampal cortex
Choroid plexus | Pyramidal layer of hippocampal cortex

547 | Granular layer of dentate gyrus

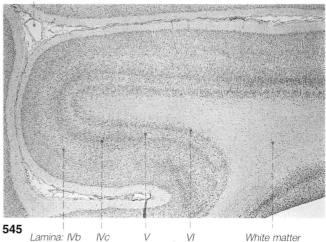

Vein in arachnoid of calcarine sulcus

545 | Lamina: IVb | IVc | V | VI | White matter

Fig. 544. Frontal section through calcarine sulcus (primary visual area) showing prominent lamination of this granular type of isocortex. Layer IV is particularly thick and subdivided by a light band into three sublayers (IVa, b and c). This lighter band contains fewer cells and is occupied by large numbers of myelinated fibers which give rise to the line of Gennari in specimens stained for myelin. Nissl staining (with toluidine blue). Magnification 6×.

Fig. 545. Close-up of the lower part of the preceding figure to illustrate lamination of visual cortex (striate area). Adjacent to the white matter lies lamina VI which is distinct because of its cellularity. Then follows a narrow lighter band (= lamina V) which borders onto a thicker and intensely staining lamina IVc. The next outward layer contains again fewer cells and hence appears lighter. This is the broad lamina IVb (= line of Gennari in sections stained for myelin) which is followed by the more cellular, yet thin lamina IVa. Laminae III and II cannot be clearly distinguished from each other but they comprise the layer between lamina IVa and the outermost nearly unstained lamina I. Nissl staining. Magnification 16×.

Fig. 546. Frontal section through hippocampal formation with dentate gyrus, hippocampus and inferior horn of the lateral ventricle containing parts of the choroid plexus. The orientation of this section is such that the medial aspect of the brain corresponds to the upper margin of this micrograph and the base lies parallel to the left margin. The dentate gyrus is easily identified by its prominent, intensely staining granular layer. Nissl staining. Magnification 6×.

Fig. 547. Close-up of the preceding micrograph shows parts of the pyramidal layer of the hippocampal cortex dissolving into a loosely arranged complex of cells that is engulfed by the granular layer of the dentate gyrus. Nissl staining. Magnification 20×.

234

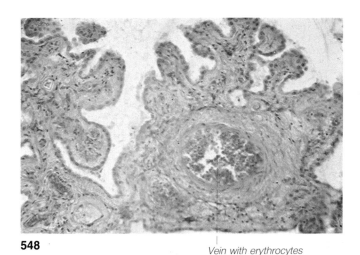

548

Vein with erythrocytes

Veins filled with erythrocytes

Figs. 548 and 549. Parts of choroid plexus from human lateral ventricle. These highly vascular folded connective tissue lamellae project into the ventricles and produce the cerebrospinal fluid (CSF). Their simple cuboidal epithelium functions as a selective barrier for materials moving from the blood into the CSF, thus forming part of the blood-CSF barrier. At higher magnification (Fig. 549) individual villi of the choroid plexus can be confused with those of the placenta (see next figure). H & E staining. Magnifications 120 × and 240 ×, respectively.

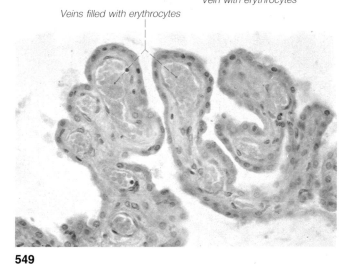

549

Surface epithelium with irregularly distributed nuclei

Fig. 550. Villus from mature human placenta (same specimen as shown in Figs. 441, 442). When compared to the foregoing choroidal villi those of the placenta are distinguishable by 1) their looser connective tissue core, 2) an irregular distribution of the nuclei within the surface epithelium (because it is a syncytium) and 3) the regular presence of fibrinoid in the intervillous space (cf. also Figs. 440, 442). H & E staining. Magnification 240 ×.

550

Fibrinoid

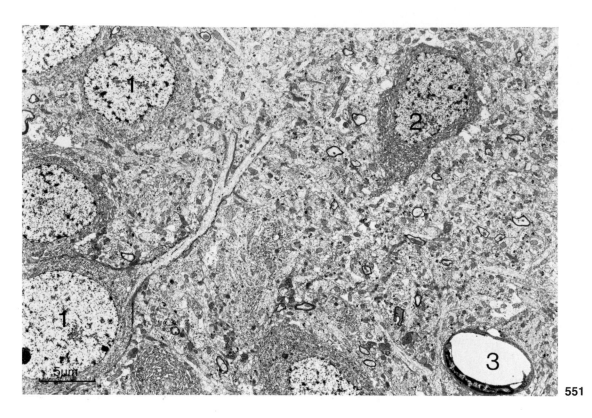

Fig. 551. Low-power electron micrograph of rat cerebral cortex illustrating several nerve cells that have small round or ovoid peri-karya containing a large vesicular nucleus (**1**). One dendrite, originating from the cell in the left lower corner, has been out-lined in black to demarcate it from the rest of the neuropil. The darker staining cone-shaped cell (**2**) is not an oligodendrocyte, but a nerve cell that shows artifactual damage. **3** Capillary lumen. Magnification 3,000×.

Fig. 552. A higher magnification of the so-called neuropil of rat cerebral cortex reveals its rather confusing complexity. The neuro-pil is all of the glial and nerve cell processes interposed between the ganglion cells and hence it consists of a multitude of variously shaped cytoplasmic profiles differing in size and structural composition. Sites of synaptic contact can be identified by an accumula-tion of vesicles within the presynaptic element and a thicker, very electron dense opposing cell membrane of the postsynaptic compo-nent (**1**). **2** Myelinated axon. Magnification 29,000×.

Fig. 553. High-power electron micrograph of several synapses of the cortical neuropil of rat motor cortex. Due to the electron lucent contents of the synaptic vesicles (**1**) their transmitter substance most probably is acetylcholine. Magnification 72,000×.

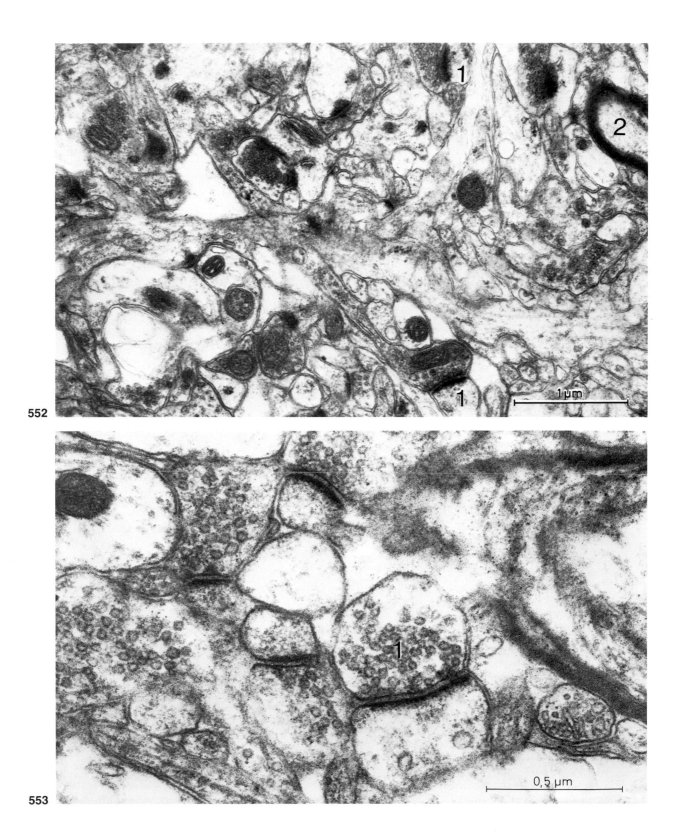

552

553

Tables

Tables

Table 1. Histologic stains

Histologic stains	Nuclei	Cytoplasm	Collagenous fibers	Elastic fibers
H & E = hematoxylin and eosin	blue-violet	red	red	unstained or light pink
Mallory-azan = azocarmine and aniline blue modified after Mallory	red	light pink or bluish	blue	unstained (but can be red or reddish blue when fibers are highly concentrated as in elastic membranes and ligaments)
Elastica stain (resorcin-fuchsin or orcein) mostly combined with nuclear fast red (counterstain)	red	light pink	grey	blackish violet or dark brown
Van Gieson (iron hematoxylin, picric acid and acid fuchsin)	black	yellow	red	no specific color (but can be yellow when fibers are highly concentrated as in elastic membranes and ligaments)
Trichrome stain after Masson-Goldner (iron hematoxylin; Ponceau acid fuchsin; azophloxine/light green)	brownish black	orange-red	green	no specific color
Iron hematoxylin after Heidenhain (particularly suitable for the staining of cell organelles, muscular cross-striations, etc.)	bluish black	—	—	light grey

240

Table 2.

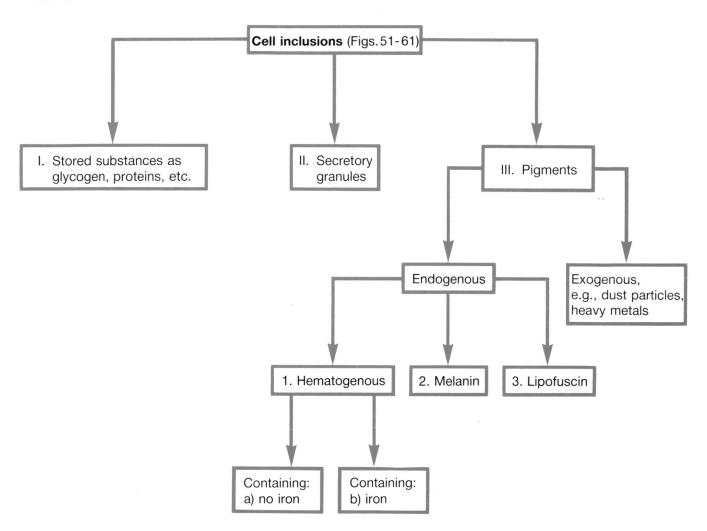

Table 3. Classification of epithelial tissues according to the shape of cells and their arrangement (after H. Petersen)

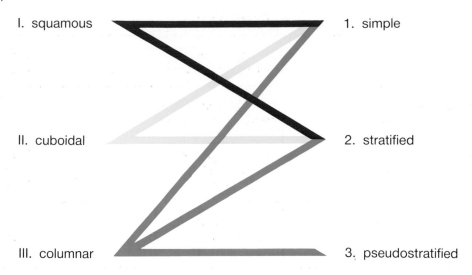

I. squamous		1. simple
II. cuboidal		2. stratified
III. columnar		3. pseudostratified

Table 4. Types of epithelial tissues and their locations

I. squamous	1. simple	predominantly all meso- and endothelia
	2. stratified	a) cornified, e.g., skin b) noncornified, e.g., oral cavity, vagina, cornea, esophagus
II. cuboidal	1. simple	e.g., in excretory ducts, some kidney tubules, germinal epithelium of the ovary, etc.
	2. stratified	transitional epithelium
III. columnar	1. simple	a) with motile cilia: uterus, uterine tube b) without motile cilia: gastrointestinal tract, gallbladder
	2. stratified	(infrequent) conjunctival fornix, parts of the male and female urethra
	3. pseudostratified	a) without motile cilia: certain parts of glandular ducts (infrequent) b) with motile cilia: respiratory tract c) with stereocilia: ductus epididymidis, ductus deferens

Table 5. Principles for the classification of exocrine glands

Morphological criteria	Classifications	Examples
1. According to the number of secretory cells	unicellular glands multicellular glands	goblet cells salivary glands
2. According to the location of the secretory cells in relation to the epithelium	intraepithelial glands extraepithelial glands	goblet cells all large exocrine glands
3. According to the mechanism of secretion	holocrine glands merocrine glands apocrine glands	sebaceous glands sweat glands prostate gland
4. According to the nature of the secretion	serous glands mucous glands mucoid glands	parotid gland goblet cells pyloric glands
5. According to the shape of the secretory units	tubular glands acinar glands alveolar glands mixed forms: tubulo-acinar glands tubulo-alveolar glands	crypts of Lieberkühn parotid gland apocrine sweat glands submandibular gland lactating mammary gland
6. According to the occurrence and the arrangement (i.e. branched or not) of a duct system	simple glands (each secretory portion empties separately on an epithelial surface) branched glands (several secretory units empty into an unbranched excretory duct) compound glands (secretory portions empty into an elaborate branched duct system)	sweat glands pyloric glands all large salivary glands

Table 6. "Family tree" of the different types of the connective tissues (modified after K. Zeiger, 1948)

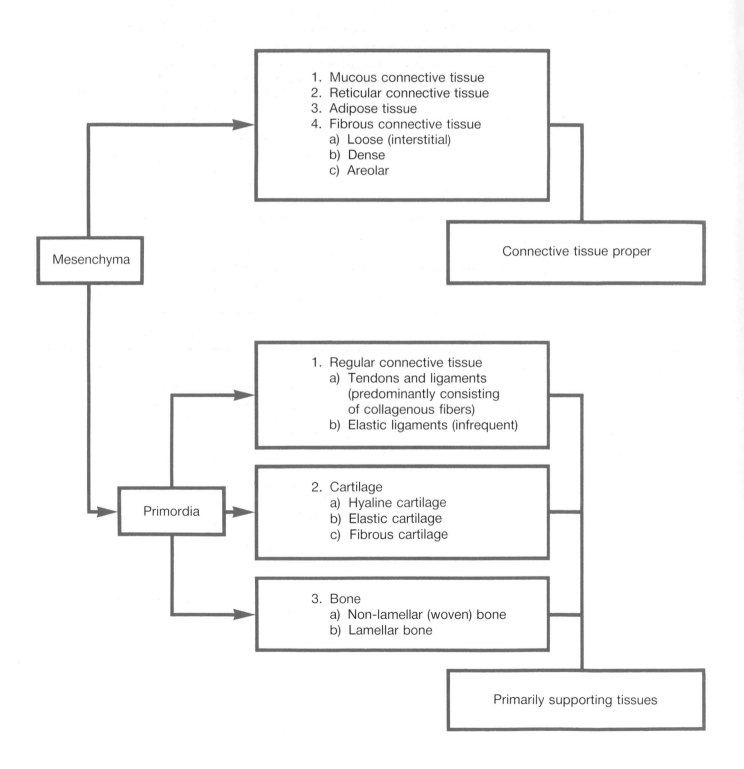

Table 7. Various biological, light microscopic and staining properties of connective tissue fibers

	Collagenous fibers	Elastic fibers	Reticular fibers
Arrangement	meshworks of varying texture	true networks or fenestrated membranes (e.g., inner elastic lamina)	delicate networks (regularly located at the interface between the interstitial connective tissue and the parenchymal cells of almost every organ)
Microscopic appearance in fresh preparations	undulating course of longitudinally striated bundles of fibrils, poorly refractile	glassy, homogeneous (no fibrillar substructure), double contoured, highly refractile	not recognizable as such
Optical properties	highly anisotropic, hence showing uniaxial form and crystalline birefringence	isotropic in an unstretched state (hence no birefringence) but with increasing distension becoming anisotropic	slightly birefringent
Behavior in dilute acids	considerable swelling	—	moderate swelling
Behavior in dilute alkalis	dissolution	—	moderate dissolution
Mechanical properties	non-extensible	reversibly extensible to about 150% of their original length	moderately extensible
Staining properties Mallory-azan	blue	unstained (but orange-red when in high concentrations as in elastic membranes)	blue
H&E	red	unstained (but light pink when in higher concentrations)	no specific color
Van Gieson	red	unstained (but yellow when in higher concentrations)	no specific color

Table 8. Various types of "fibers"

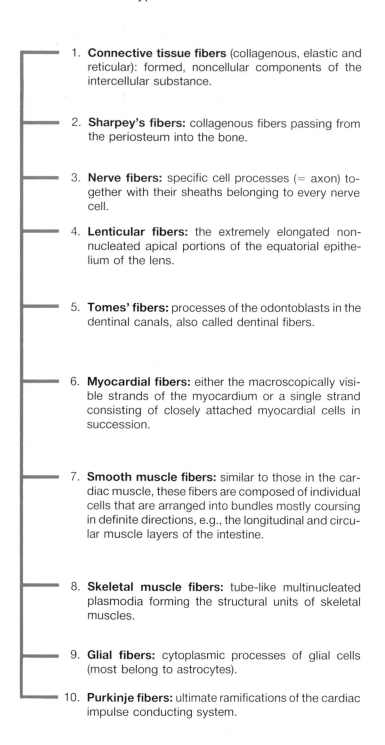

1. **Connective tissue fibers** (collagenous, elastic and reticular): formed, noncellular components of the intercellular substance.

2. **Sharpey's fibers:** collagenous fibers passing from the periosteum into the bone.

3. **Nerve fibers:** specific cell processes (= axon) together with their sheaths belonging to every nerve cell.

4. **Lenticular fibers:** the extremely elongated non-nucleated apical portions of the equatorial epithelium of the lens.

5. **Tomes' fibers:** processes of the odontoblasts in the dentinal canals, also called dentinal fibers.

6. **Myocardial fibers:** either the macroscopically visible strands of the myocardium or a single strand consisting of closely attached myocardial cells in succession.

7. **Smooth muscle fibers:** similar to those in the cardiac muscle, these fibers are composed of individual cells that are arranged into bundles mostly coursing in definite directions, e.g., the longitudinal and circular muscle layers of the intestine.

8. **Skeletal muscle fibers:** tube-like multinucleated plasmodia forming the structural units of skeletal muscles.

9. **Glial fibers:** cytoplasmic processes of glial cells (most belong to astrocytes).

10. **Purkinje fibers:** ultimate ramifications of the cardiac impulse conducting system.

Table 9. Easily recognizable essential features for the differentiation of muscular tissues

Type of tissue	Structural unit	Number of nuclei per structural unit	Location of the nuclei	Shape of the nuclei	Size of the structural units	
					length	diameter
Skeletal muscle	fiber	several hundreds up to thousands	subsarcolemmal	elongated, flat	up to several cm	20–100 μm
Myocardium	cell	1–2	central, with perinuclear cytoplasm free of myofibrils	plumpish round-ovoid	50–120 μm	10–20 μm
Smooth muscle	cell	1	central	elongated, rod-shaped or elliptical	40–200 μm (in a pregnant uterus up to 500 μm)	5–10 μm

Table 10. Histologic characteristics useful for identifying lymphoid organs

	Tonsils	Lymph node	Thymus	Spleen
Epithelium	+	−	−	−
Connective tissue capsule	−	+	+	+
Organization into cortex and medulla	−	+	+	−
Marginal sinus	−	+	−	−
Hassall's corpuscles	−	−	+	−
Malpighian bodies	−	−	−	+

Tables

Table 11. Compilation of those regions that possess several surfaces usually covered by different epithelia

	Lips	Uvula	Epiglottis	Eyelids	Nostrils	Ear lobes	Uterine cervix
Epithelium changes from:	Epidermis with hairs and various glands to the squamous, stratified and noncornified variety	Stratified squamous noncornified to a pseudo-stratified, columnar and ciliated epithelium	Stratified squamous noncornified to a pseudo-stratified, columnar and ciliated epithelium	Epidermis (without hair follicles) to a stratified, noncornified squamous epithelium	Epidermis with seba-ceous glands unconnected with hairs to an epidermal epithelium with hairs (vibrissae) and glands followed by a respiratory epithelium	Both surfaces are covered by the same epithelium: epidermis with typical cutaneous adnexes	Stratified noncornified squamous epithelium (covering the outer sur-face) to a sim-ple columnar epithelium (lining the cervical canal)
Central tissue core predominantly consisting of:	Skeletal muscle (orbicularis oris muscle)	Skeletal muscle (uvular muscle)	Elastic cartilage	Skeletal muscle (orbicularis oculi muscle) and Meibo-mian glands	Hyaline cartilage	Elastic cartilage	Smooth muscle

248

Table 12. Differentiation of the salivary glands, the lacrimal gland, and the exocrine pancreas

Gland	Shape of secretory units	Duct system	Other characteristics
Parotid	Acinar (serous)	Elaborate, conspicuous, large numbers of striated ducts (best criterion to distinguish parotid gland from exocrine pancreas)	Numerous fat cells together with sections of the arborizations of the facial nerve
Sub-mandibular	Tubulo-acinar (sero-mucous) with a prevailing serous (acinar) component	Well developed	Serous demilunes capping the tubular (mucous) secretory units
Sublingual	Tubulo-acinar (sero-mucous) with a prevailing mucous (tubular) component	Intercalated and striated (salivary) ducts are sparse	Serous demilunes capping the tubular (mucous) secretory units
Lacrimal	Tubulo-alveolar	No intercalated or striated ducts, therefore a "branched" gland	Serous (!) secretion. In the connective tissue septa aggregations of free cells, especially plasma cells
Exocrine pancreas	Acinar (serous)	No striated ducts, rest of the duct system much less developed than in parotid gland	Centro-acinar cells

Tables

Table 13. Differentiation of the consecutive segments of the digestive tract, including the gallbladder

Part of the digestive tract	Folds	Villi	Crypts	Goblet cells	Special characteristics
Stomach, fundus	Sparse and coarse	−	−	−	Shallow gastric pits, deep fundic glands with chief and parietal cells
Stomach, pyloric part	Rare and coarse	−	−	−	Deep gastric pits, low pyloric glands, no chief or parietal cells
Duodenum	Elaborate	+	+	+	Glands of Brunner within the submucosa, including that of the folds
Jejunum	Numerous	+	+	+	
Ileum	Decreasing in number and lower	+	+	+	Aggregated lymphoid nodules (Peyer's patches) within the submucosa
Colon	Rare and coarse	−	+	+	Mucosa contains crypts but no villi
Vermiform appendix	−	−	+	+	Large focal lymphoid aggregates within the submucosa and the mucosa
Gallbladder	Very delicate anastomosing folds	−	−	−	No layering of the muscular tunic (characteristic criterion for differentiation)

Table 14. Differentiation of various "alveolar" glands and the fetal lung

Gland	Lobular subdivisions	Duct system	Secretory units	Special characteristics
Prostate	Poorly defined	Almost nonexistent	Wide alveoli with a frill-like inner contour	Interstitial connective tissue packed with smooth muscle (crucial criterion for diagnosis)
Lactating mammary	Very distinct	Excretory ducts are regularly seen in the interlobular septa (crucial criterion for diagnosis)	Varying in size, lipid vacuoles within the secretory cells	
Thyroid	Distinct	None	Follicles are the largest of all alveolar secretory units, size and lumen vary	"Secretory units" (= follicles) filled with deeply staining material (colloid)
Fetal lung	Distinct, conspicuous cellular connective tissue	Always distinct	Often appearing as branching epithelial tubules	Close to the "duct" system (primordia of bronchi) hyaline cartilage can be found (crucial criterion for diagnosis)

Table 15. Differentiation of hollow organs showing a stellate lumen in cross-section

Organ	Epithelium	Muscular tunic	Special characteristics
Esophagus	Squamous, stratified noncornified	Very prominent, distinctly divided into inner circular and outer longitudinal layer	Prominent muscularis mucosae, scattered small glands within the submucosa
Ureter	Transitional	More loosely arranged, subdivided into a prominent intermediate circular layer to which inner and outer bundles of longitudinal muscles are loosely attached	
Urethra	Columnar, bi- to four-layered, pseudostratified or stratified	No distinct layering, very loosely arranged muscular network	Prominent venous plexus within the lamina propria
Ductus deferens	Columnar, pseudostratified with stereocilia	Very prominent, distinctly arranged into inner longitudinal, intermediate circular and outer longitudinal layer	Often sectioned together with the entire spermatic cord
Uterine tube	Columnar, simple with motile cilia	Relatively thick, no distinct layering, preferentially circular	Slender, richly arborized mucosal folds

Subject Index

Index

Index

Index

Index

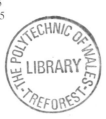